GLOSSARY OF MEDICAL,
HEALTH AND PHARMACY TERMS
FRENCH-ENGLISH and ENGLISH-FRENCH

GLOSSAIRE DES TERMES MÉDICAUX,
DE SANTÉ ET DE PHARMACIE
FRANÇAIS-ANGLAIS et ANGLAIS-FRANÇAIS

compiled by

ALAN S. LINDSEY

HADLEY PAGER INFO

First Edition, 2003

ISBN 1-872739-12-1

Reprinted August 2003

Printed and bound in England by Ralph Wrightson Ltd.,
Earls Barton

HADLEY PAGER INFO
Leatherhead, Surrey, England

FOREWORD

The Glossary is a completely new compilation providing an up-to-date source of over 3000 medical, health and pharmacy terms in both French and English. It covers a wide range of illnesses and diseases, as well as anatomical terms, first-aid and hospital terms, together with pharmacy terms embracing medicines, toiletries, cosmetics, health and pharmaceutical products.

A large number of the more technical terms are provided with brief aide-memoire (AM) definitions in English and French, but users are recommended to get a suitable handbook in their own native language to obtain detailed knowledge of the various medical terms, for example in English the Mosby Nurses Pocket Dictionary published by Harcourt Publishers or in French the Dictionnaire Médical de Poche published by Masson, Paris.

Many phrases in French and English are included which can be used in medical situations. The Glossary should be of value to English speakers visiting or living in French speaking regions and to French speakers visiting or living in English speaking regions. A visit to a Pharmacie in France or a Chemist's Shop in Britain will usually help in tracking down the address of a local doctor, dentist or hospital.

I am greatly indebted to my wife, Hazel Lindsey, for her considerable assistance in the preparation of the text, as well as with the proof-reading. I would ask users of the Glossary to let me know of any errors or omissions that they might note so that these can be rectified in later editions.

It should be noted that translations given in the Glossary are those generally recognised but they have no legal, statutory or official basis. Terms which the compiler has reason to believe are registered trade names or marks are indicated by the symbol ®. However, the presence or absence of such a symbol should not be regarded as affecting the legal status of any trade mark or name.

A.S.L.

Abbreviations Used

adj	adjective	*prep*	preposition or	AM	aide-memoire
adv	adverb		prepositional	ant	antonym
f	feminine noun		phrase	colloq	colloquial
m	masculine noun	*pron*	pronoun	cosmet	cosmetic
inv	invariant	*pp*	past participle	eg	for example
conj	conjunction	*v*	verb	nom pop	nom populaire
pl	plural			par ex	par exemple
		®	registered trade	syn	synonym
			mark	terme mod	terme moderne
				US	United States of America

abasie *f* [AM: incapacité de marcher]   abasia [AM: motor incoordination in walking]

abcès *m*   abscess
- abcès à la gencive = gumboil
- j'ai un abcès = I have an abscess
- vider un abcès = to drain an abscess

abdomen *m*   abdomen

abdominal,-e *adj*   abdominal

abdominaux *mpl*   abdominal muscles; stomach muscles
- faire des abdominaux = to exercise the stomach muscles

abducteur *m* ; **also** *adj*   abductor muscle

abduction *f*   abduction

aberration *f*   aberration

aberration *f* **chromosomique**   chromosomic aberration

aberration *f* **sphérique**   spherical aberration

abimer *v*   to damage (eg hands)
- hépatite peut abîmer le foie = hepatitis can damage the liver

ablation *f* **chirurgicale**   surgical removal (of an organ)

absorption *f*   absorption

acarien *m*   acarid; tick; mite

accès *m*   seizure, fit; attack
- accès de fièvre = attack/bout of fever
- accès de toux = attack of coughing

accident *m*   accident
- accident cardio-vasculaire = cardiovascular accident
- accident vasculaire cérébral (syn. infarctus cérébral) = stroke; cerebrovascular accident

accouchement *m*   childbirth; delivery
- accouchement à terme/ avant terme = full term/premature birth
- accouchement difficile/facile = a difficult/an easy birth/delivery
- accouchement par le siège; siège *m* = breech birth; breech delivery
- accouchement provoqué = induced delivery

accoucher *v*   to deliver (a child); to give birth
- accoucher de = to give birth to

accoucheuse *f*   midwife; obstetrician

acide *m* **acétylsalicylique**   acetyl salicylic acid (aspirin)

acide *m* **ascorbique**   ascorbic acid (vitamin C)

acide *m* **borique**   boric acid

acide *m* **citrique**   citric acid

acide *m* **folique**   folic acid

acide *m* **ribonucléique**   ribonucleic acid

acide *m* urique uric acid
acides *mpl* gras fatty acids
- les acides gras insaturés = unsaturated fatty acids
- les acides gras monoinsaturés = monounsaturated fatty acids
- les acides gras polyinsaturés = polyunsaturated fatty acids
- les acides gras saturés = saturated fatty acids

acidité *f* acidity
acidité *f* gastrique gastric acidity
acidose *f* acidosis
acné *f* acne
acné *f* rosacée; rosacée acne rosacea
acoumétrie *f* [AM: evaluation de l'acuité auditive] acoumetry [AM: evaluation of hearing]
acouphène *m* tinnitus aurium (ear)
acquis,-ise *adj* acquired
- caractère acquis = acquired character
- immunité acquise = acquired immunity

acromégalie *f* [AM: maladie rare, provoquant augmentation des mains, de la tête etc]
  acromegaly [AM: rare disease causing enlargement of hands, face etc.]
acuité *f* acuity; acuteness
acupuncture *f* acupuncture
adducteur *m*; also *adj* adductor muscle
adduction *f* adduction
adénite *f* [AM: inflammation d'un ganglion lymphatique] adenitis [AM: inflammation of a lymphatic ganglion]
adénome *m* [AM: tumeur bénigne sur une glande] adenoma [AM: benign tumour on a gland]
adhérence *f* adhesion
adolescence *f* adolescence
adolescent,-e *adj* adolescent
adolescent *m*; adolescente *f* adolescent
adoucissant *m*; adoucissant,-ante *adj* demulcent; softener
adrénaline *f* adrenaline; epinephrine
adulte *m,f* adult
aérobic *m* aerobics
aérocolie *f* aerocoly
aérogastrie *f* aerogastria
aérophagie *f* aerophagy
aérosol *m* aerosol
affection *f* 1 disease; 2 affection
- affection hépatique = biliousness
- affection respiratoire = respiratory affection

- affections congénitales = congenital ailments/diseases

aftershave *m* aftershave

âge *m* age
- âge bas; petite enfance *f* = infancy
- âge mental = mental age
- âge préscolaire = preschool age
- âge (troisième); les personnes âgées = elderly
- âges, entre deux = middle-aged
- quel âge avez-vous? = how old are you?; what is your age?

agent *m* **coagulant du sang** blood clotting agent

agent *m* **thérapeutique** medicine; remedy; cure

agglutination *f* agglutination; clumping

agglutiner *v* to agglutinate

agglutinine *f* agglutinin

agrafe *f* clip; agraffe

aigreurs *fpl* **d'estomac** heartburn; stomach acid

aide-soignant *m*; **aide-soignante** *f* nursing auxiliary; nurse's aide

aigu, aiguë *adj* acute; sharp
- douleur aiguë = sharp pain
- maladie aigüe de l'appareil respiratoire = acute respiratory disease

aiguille *f* needle (eg of syringe)

aiguille *f* **pour injections** hypodermic needle

aine *f* groin

aisselle *f* armpit; axilla

albinisme *m* albinism

albumine *f* albumin

albuminurie *f* albuminuria

alcaloïde *m* alkaloid

alcool *m* alcohol
- alcool à 90 (degrés); alcool modifié à 90 = surgical spirit
- alcool absolu = pure alcohol; absolute alcohol

alcoolémie *f* presence of alcohol in the blood
- contrôle d'alcoolémie = checking for alcohol in the blood
- taux d'alcoolémie = level of alcohol in the blood

alcoolisme *m* alcoholism

Alcootest ® *m* Breathalyser (instrument)
- faire subir l'Alcootest à = to breathalyse

alcootest *m* breathalyser test

aliments pour bébés; alimentation *f* **pour bébé** baby food

allaitement *m* **artificiel** bottle feeding

allaitement *m* **maternel** breast-feeding

allaitement *m* **mixte**   mixed feeding
allaiter *v*   to breastfeed
- allaiter au biberon = to bottle feed
- j'allaite mon enfant = I'm breastfeeding
allergène *m*   allergen
allergie *f*   allergy
- allergie cutanée = skin allergy
- allergie de contact = contact allergy
- allergie respiratoire = respiratory allergy
allergique *adj* (à)   allergic (to)
- je suis allergique à la pénicilline
allopathie *f* [AM: méthode thérapeutique]   allopathy [AM: therapeutic method]
alopécie *f* [AM: chute des cheveux]   alopecia [AM: hair loss]
alphabloquant *m*   alpha-blocker; alpha-blocking
alvéolite *f* **pulmonaire**   alveolitis (of the lungs)
Alzheimer, maladie d' [AM: dégénérescence cérébrale]   Alzheimer's disease [AM: degeneration of the brain cortex]
amalgame m **dentaire**   dental amalgam
ambulance *f*   ambulance
ambulatoire *adj*   ambulatory
- malade ambulatoire = ambulatory patient
- traitement ambulatoire = ambulatory care
aménorrhée *f* [AM: absence des règles]   amenorrhoea [AM: absence of menstruation]
amibe *f* [AM: parasite bactérien]   amoeba; ameba [AM: parasitic bacterium]
amincir (s') *v*   to get slimmer
amincissant,-e *adj*   slimming
- produit amincissant = slimming product
amincissement *m*   slimming
ammoniaque *f*   ammonia
amnésie *f*   amnesia
amniocentèse *f*   amniocentesis
amniotique *adj*   amniotic
- cavité *f* amniotique = amniotic cavity
- liquide *m* amniotique = amniotic fluid
- poche *f* des eaux = amniotic sac
amphétamine *f*   amphetamine
ampoule *f*   1 blister; 2 ampulla; 3 phial; ampoule
- ampoule rectale = rectal ampulla
- couvert d'ampoules = blistered
- pansement pour l'ampoule = blister plaster
- se couvrir d'ampoules = to blister

amputation *f* amputation

amygdalectomie *f* (syn. tonsillectomie) [AM: ablation des amygdales] tonsillectomy [AM: tonsil removal]

amygdales *fpl* tonsils

amygdalite *f* tonsillitis

anabolisant *m* stéroïdien; anabolisant *m*; also *adj* anabolic steroid

anal,-e *adj* anal

analgésie *f* analgesia

analgésique *m*; also *adj* analgesic; painkiller; anodyne

analyse *f* analysis
- analyse de sang = blood test; blood examination
- analyse d'urine = urine analysis

anaphylactique *adj* anaphylactic
- choc anaphylactique = anaphylactic shock

anaphylaxie *f* anaphylaxy; anaphylaxis

anasarque *f* [AM: œdème généralisé du tissu] anasarca [AM: general oedema of the tissues]

anatomie *f* anatomy

anatomique *adj* anatomical

androgène *m* androgen (male hormone)

andropause *f* male menopause; male climacteric

androstérone *f* androsterone (male hormone)

anémie *f* anaemia
- anémie/maladie de Biermer = pernicious anaemia
- anémie pernicieuse = pernicious anaemia

anémie pernicieuse progressive *f* pernicious anaemia

anémique *adj* anaemic

anesthésie *f* anesthesia; anaesthesia
- anesthésie épidurale = epidural anesthesia
- anesthésie générale = general anesthesia
- anesthésie locale = local anesthesia
- anesthésie péridurale = peridural anesthesia
- faire une anesthésie locale/générale = to give someone a local/general anaesthetic

anesthésier *v* to anesthetize; to anaesthetize; to block (pain)

anesthésique *m*; also *adj* anaesthetic; anesthesic
- agent anesthésique = anaesthetic

anesthésiste *m,f* anesthetist; anaesthetist

anévrisme *m* aneurism; aneurysm
- anévrisme artériel = arterial aneurism

angéite *f* angeitis

antidiurétique

angine *f* throat infection; tonsillitis; pharyngitis; angina
- angine de poitrine = angina pectoris
- angine de Vincent = Vincent's angina/disease
- angine rouge = tonsillitis
- avoir une angine = to have a sore throat

angiocardiographie *f* [AM: examen aux rayons X du cœur] angiocardiography [AM: x-ray examination of heart]

angiographie *f* angiography

angiome *m* [AM: tumeur formée par agglomération de vaisseaux sanguins] angioma [AM: tumour composed of blood vessels]

angoisse *f* anxiety; distress; angor; spasm

angor *m* angina pectoris

ankylose *f* [AM: limitation de la mobilité d'une articulation] ankylosis [AM: part or total immobility of a joint]

ankylostome *m* hookworm

ankylostomiase *f*; **ankylostomose** *f* hookworm disease; ankylostomiasis; uncinariasis

anneau *m* **de dentition** teething ring

annulaire *m* third finger

anorexie *f* anorexia
- anorexie mentale = anorexia nervosa

anormal *adj* anomalous

anthrax *m* anthrax

antiacide *m; also adj* antacid

antiacnéique *m* cream, gel etc. for treatment of acne

anti-âge *adj* **(prévention)** prevention of ageing

antiagrégant plaquettaire anti (blood) platelet aggregation

antiallergique *adj* allergy alleviating

antiarthritique *m; also adj* drug etc. alleviating arthritis

antiasthmatique *m; also adj* drug etc. alleviating asthma

antibactérien,-ienne *adj* antibacterial

antibotique *m; also adj* antibiotic
- être sous antibiotiques = to be on antibiotics

anticancéreux,-euse *adj* antineoplastic; anticancer (eg treatment)
- centre anticancéreux = cancer hospital
- sérum anticancéreux = cancer serum

anticoagulant *m; also adj* anticoagulant

anticonceptionnel *m; also adj* contraceptive

anticorps *m* antibody

antidépresseur *m*; **antidépressif** *m; also adj* antidepressant

antidiurétique *m; also adj* antidiuretic

antidote *m* antidote
antidouleur *adj* pain relieving; analgesic
antifongique *m; also adj* antifungal
antigène *m* antigen
antigénique *adj* antigenic
antihelminthique *m; also adj* [AM: médicament pour l'élimination des vers intestinaux]
  anthelmintic; antihelminthic [AM: remedy for eliminating intestinal worms]
antihistaminique *m; also adj* antihistamine
  ▪ produit m antihistaminique = antihistamine
anti-inflammatoire *adj* anti-inflammatory
antioxydant *m; also adj* antioxidant
antipyrétique *m; also adj* antipyretic; febrifuge
antiscorbutique *adj* antiscorbutic
antisepsie *f* antisepsis
antiseptique *m; also adj* antiseptic
antispasmodique *m; also adj* antispasmodic (eg drug)
antitoxine *f* antitoxin
antitoxique *adj* antitoxic
antitussif *m* cough mixture; cough syrup
antitussif *m;* **antitussif,-ive** *adj* antitussive
antiviral,-e *adj* antiviral
anurèse *f* anuresis; anuria
anurie *f* anuresis; anuria
anus *m* anus
anxiété *f* anxiety
aorte *f* aorta
apaisant,-e *adj* soothing
  ▪ crème/lotion/poudre apaisante = soothing cream/lotion/powder
aphasie *f* [AM: incapacité de parler qui est due à une atteinte cérébrale] aphasia [AM:
  inability to speak due to brain disease or injury]
aphonie *f* [AM: extinction de voix] aphonia [AM: loss of voice]
aphrodisiaque *m* aphrodisiac
aphte *m* mouth ulcer; aphta
aponévrite *f* fibrositis
apophyse *f* [AM: saillie osseuse] apophysis; process [AM: bony outgrowth]
apoplectique *adj* apoplectic
  ▪ attaque f d'apoplexie = apoplectic fit
apoplexie *f* apoplexy; stroke
  ▪ attaque f d'apoplexie = to have a stroke
appareil *m* **acoustique** hearing aid; deaf-aid
appareil *m* **dentaire; appareil orthodontique** brace(s) (for teeth)

appareil digestif digestive system
appareil *m* **lacrymal** lachrymal apparatus
appareil *m* **orthopédique** brace
appareil *m* **respiratoire** respiratory system
appendice *m* appendix
appendicectomie *f* [AM: ablation de l'appendice] appendicectomy; appendectomy
[AM: removal of appendix]
appendicite *f* appendicitis
  ▪ appendicite aiguë = acute appendicitis
appétit *m* appetite
  ▪ coupe-faim *m inv* = appetite depressant
  ▪ perdre l'appétit = to lose one's appetite
appliquer *v* to apply (eg ointment, dressing)
après-shampooing *m* hair conditioner
aromathérapie *f* aromatherapy
arracher *v* to extract; to pull out (eg tooth)
  ▪ je ne voudrais pas me le faire arracher = I don't want it (tooth) extracted
arrêt cardiaque cardiac arrest
artère *f* artery
  ▪ artère carotide = carotid artery
  ▪ artère cubitale = cubital artery
  ▪ artère faciale = facial artery
  ▪ artère fémorale = femoral artery
  ▪ artère humérale = humeral artery
  ▪ artère iliaque = iliac artery
  ▪ artère pédieuse = pedal artery
  ▪ artère pulmonaire = pulmonary artery
  ▪ artère radiale = radial artery
  ▪ artère sous-clavière = subclavian artery
  ▪ artère tibiale = tibial artery
arthrite *f* arthritis
  ▪ arthrite chronique juvénile; (syn: maladie de Still) = juvenile rheumatoid arthritis
  ▪ arthrite sèche déformante; arthrite chronique dégénérative; arthrose = arthritis;
    osteoarthritis
arthrose *f* osteoarthritis; degenerative joint disease
  ▪ arthrose du genou = osteoarthritis of the knee
articulation *f* joint
  ▪ articulation coxo-fémorale; articulation de la hanche = hip joint; coxa
  ▪ articulation du poignet = wrist joint
artériosclérose *f* arteriosclerosis
asbestose *f* asbestosis

ascaride *m* roundworm
ascite *f* ascites
asphyxie *f* asphyxia
aspirine *f* aspirin
  ■ aspirine soluble = soluble aspirin
  ■ je suis allergique à l'aspirine = i am allergic to aspirin
assurance *m* **maladie** health insurance; sickness benefit
asthénie *f* [AM: diminution des forces; débilité] asthenia [AM: diminution of strength; debility]
asthénique *adj* asthenic
asthmatique *adj* asthmatic
  ■ je suis asthmatique = I am asthmatic
asthme *m* asthma
astigmatisme *m* astigmatism (of eye)
astragale *m* astragalus; talus, anklebone
astringent *m*; **also** *adj* astringent
  ■ lotion astringente = astringent lotion
ataxie *f* ataxia
  ■ ataxie locomotrice = locomotor ataxia
atrophie *f* [AM: diminution de poids ou de volume d'un organe] atrophy [AM: loss of weight or volume of an organ]
atrophier *v* to atrophy
atropine *f* atropine
attaque de panique panic attack
atteindre *v* to affect; to reach
atteint,-e *adj* affected
  ■ être atteint d'une maladie = to be suffering from an illness
attelle *f* splint
attestation *f* **médicale** medical certificate
audiogram *m* audiogram
audiomètre *m* audiometer
audiométrie *f* [AM: mesure instrumentale de l'audition] audiometry [AM: instrumental measurement of hearing]
audiophone *m*; **audiphone** *m* hearing aid
audition *f* hearing; audition
auriculaire *adj* auricular (ear, heart)
auriculaire *m* little finger
autisme *m* autism
autiste *m,f* autistic person
autiste *adj* autistic
autistique *adj* autistic

bandage

auto-immunité *f* auto-immunity
autoclave *m* [AM: appareil utilisé pour la stérilisation par la vapeur] autoclave [AM: appliance used for steam sterilization]
autogène *adj* autogenous; autogenic
auto-intoxication *f* (syn. **autotoxicose; autotoxémie**) auto-intoxication
autolyse *f* autolysis
automatisme *m* automatism
autoplastie *f* autoplasty
autopsie *f* autopsy
autosuggestion *f* autosuggestion
autotoxine *f* autotoxin
auxiliaire *m,f* **médicale** paramedic
avaler *v* to swallow
  ▪ ne pas avaler = not to be taken internally
avant-bras *m* forearm
aveugle *m,f* blind man/woman
avortement *m* abortion
  ▪ se faire avorter = to have an abortion
avortement *m* **spontané** miscarriage
avorter *v* to abort
  ▪ faire avorter = to abort
avulsion *f* **dentaire** tooth extraction

B

bacille *m* bacillus
bactéricide *m*; **also** *adj* bactericide
bactérie *f*; **bactéries** *fpl* bacterium; bacteria *(pl)*
bactérien,-ienne *adj* bacterial
bactériologie *f* bacteriology
bactériologique *adj* bacteriological
bactériologiste *m,f* bacteriologist
bain *m* **de boue** mud bath
bain *m* **de paraffine** wax bath
balanite *f* [AM: inflammation du gland de la verge] balanitis [AM: inflammation of the glans penis]
ballonnement *m* bloating; distension (of stomach)
bandage *m* bandage (prepared dressing)

16

- bandage herniaire = truss
- bandage mécanique = truss
- bandage triangulaire = triangular bandage
- faire un bandage à quelqu'un = to bandage someone up

bande *f* bandage
- bande de gaze = gauze roller bandage
- bande de tissu élastique = elastic support bandage
- bande elastique = elastique bandage
- bande plâtrée = plaster bandage

bandelette *f* small bandage

bander *v* to bandage

banque *f* bank
- banque de peau = skin bank
- banque de plasma = plasma bank
- banque de sang = blood bank
- banque de sperme = sperm bank

barbiturique *m* barbiturate

barrette *f* hairclip

bassin *m* pelvis
- petit bassin = lower pelvis

bassin *m* **de lit** bedpan

bassin *m* **(hygiénique)** bedpan

bavoir *m* bib (baby's)

bébé *m* baby
- attendre un bébé = to be expecting a baby

bec-de-lièvre *m* harelip

bégaiment *m* stammering; stuttering

belladone *f* belladonna

bénin, bénigne *adj* (ant. malin, maligne) benign
- tumeur bénigne = benign tumour

béquille *f* **commune** underarm crutch

béquille *f* **d'avant-bras** forearm crutch

bêtabloquant *m*; **bêtabloqueur** *m* beta-blocker; beta-blocking

biberon *m* baby's bottle
- nourir au biberon = to bottle feed

bicarbonate *m* **de sodium** sodium bicarbonate

biceps *m* biceps (muscles)

bien-être *m* wellbeing; welfare

bigoudi *m* hair curler

bilan *m* **de santé** health check-up

bile *f* bile

bilharziose *f* **(syn. schistosomiase)** [AM: infestation par vers (bilharzies)] bilharzia;
bilharziasis [AM: infestation by worms (bilharzia)]
bilieux,-ieuse *adj* bilious
bilirubine *f* bilirubin
biliverdine *f* biliverdin
biochimie *f* biochemistry
biodégradabilité *f* biodegradability
biodégradable *adj* biodegradable
biologie *f* biology
biopsie *f* biopsy
biorythme *m* biorhythm
biscuit *m* **pour bébés** rusk
blaireau *m* shaving brush
blennorragie *f* gonorrhea; gonococcal urethritis
blépharite *f* [AM: inflammation des paupières] blepharitis [AM: inflammation of the eyelids]
blessé *m*; **blessée** *f*; also *adj* injured person; casualty; injured; wounded
  ▪ blessé grave = seriously/ severely injured or wounded person
blesser *v* to injure; to make sore
blesser (se) *v* to injure oneself; to hurt oneself
blessure *f* wound; injury
bleu *m* 1 bruise; 2 blue
bleu *m* **de méthylène** [AM: colorant bleu utilisé comme antiseptique] methylene blue
  [AM: blue dye used as antiseptic]
bloc *m* block
  ▪ bloc cardiaque; bloc auriculo-ventriculaire = cardiac block
  ▪ bloc opératoire = operating suite
blocage *m* blockage; blocking
blocage *m* **articulaire** joint blocking
blocage *m* **intestinal** intestinal blockage
blush *m* blusher (cosmet)
boîte *f* **crânienne** skull
bol *m* bolus; pellet
bombe *f* **(aérosol)** spray can; arerosol can
  ▪ bombe à raser = can (aerosol) of shaving cream
bosse *f* 1 lump; 2 bump
botulisme *m* [AM: intoxication alimentaire provoquée par le bacille C.botulinum] botulism
  [AM: food poisoning due to toxin of the bacillus C.botulinum]
bouche *f* mouth
  ▪ ouvrez la bouche; tirez la langue = open your mouth; put your tongue out
bouche-à-bouche *m* mouth to mouth resuscitation
bouffée *f* **de chaleur** hot flush

bouffée *f* **délirante** period of hallucination
bouillie *f* **de sulfate de baryum** barium meal (prior to x-ray)
bouillotte *f* hot-water bottle
boulimie *f* bulimia; bulimia nervosa
bourdonnement *m* ringing (in ears); buzzing
  ▪ bourdonnement d'oreilles = ringing in the ears
bourse *f* **séreuse; bourse** *f* **synoviale** bursa
bourses *fpl* **(syn. scrotum)** scrotum
bouton *m* spot; pimple
  ▪ bouton d'acné = acne
  ▪ bouton de fièvre = cold sore
bouttonneux,-euse *adj* pimply
brancard *m* stretcher
brancardier *m* stretcher-bearer
bras *m* arm
  ▪ mon bras est cassé = my arm is broken
brillant *m* **à lèvres (cosmet)** lip gloss
brochage *m* pinning (eg a fractured bone)
broche *f* pin
bronche *f* **droite/gauche** right/left bronchus
bronchiole *f* bronchiole
bronchique *adj* bronchial
bronchite *f* bronchitis
broncho-pneumonie *f* bronchopneumonia
bronchodilatateur *m* bronchodilator
bronzage *m* sun-tanning; tan
brosse *f* **à cheveux** hairbrush
brosse *f* **à dents** toothbrush
brosse *f* **à ongles** nailbrush
brucellose *f* brucellosis; undulant fever; Malta fever
brûlure *f* burn
  ▪ brûlure du premier/deuxième/troisième degré = first/second/third degree burn
  ▪ brûlures d'estomac = heartburn
brutal,-e *adj* sudden; violent
  ▪ une obstruction brutale d'une artère coronaire = a sudden obstruction of a coronary artery
buccal,-e *adj* buccal; mouth
bulbe *m* **rachidien** spinal bulb
bulle *f* **dermatologique** dermatological bulla; large skin blister
bursite *f* bursitis

C

cabinet *m* **de consultation**   consulting room
cabinet *m* **médical**   surgery
cachet *m*   tablet
- cachet à croquer = chewable tablet
- cachet d'aspirine = aspirin tablet
- cachet soluble = soluble tablet
- prenez deux cachets par jour après les repas = take two tablets a day after meals

cadre *m* **de marche**   walking frame; walker
caecum *m*   [AM: partie de gros intestin]   caecum   [AM: part of large intestine]
cage *f* **thoracique**   thoracic cage; rib cage
caillot *m* **sanguin; caillot** *m* **de sang**   clot; blood clot
- une thrombose = a thrombosis

caissons, maladie *f* **des**   decompression sickness
cal *m*   callus
calamine *f*   calamine
- lotion calmante à la calamine = calamine lotion

calcanéum *m*   [AM: os de talon]   calcaneum   [AM: heel bone]
calcification *f*   calcification
calcium *m*   calcium
calcul *m*   calculus; stone (eg in bladder, gall bladder)
- calcul biliaire = gall stone; bile stone
- calcul rénal = kidney stone

callosité *f*   callus
calmant *m*   calmative; sedative; tranquillizer
calmant *m* **analgésique**   painkiller; analgesic
calmant *m* **pour coliques infantiles**   gripe water
calmer *v*   1 to calm down; 2 to ease; to relieve (eg pain); 3 to bring down (eg fever)
calorie *f*   calorie (heat unit)
calotte *f* **crânienne**   dome of the skull; calvarium
calvitie *f*   baldness
canal *m*   canal; duct
- canal anal = anal canal; rectum
- canal biliaire = bile duct
- canal carpien = carpal canal
- canal déférent = vas deferens
- canal thoracique = thoracic duct

cancer *m*   cancer
- cancer de la peau = skin cancer

- cancer de l'estomac = cancer of the stomach
- cancer de l'œsophage = cancer of the oesophagus
- cancer du col de l'utérus = cervical cancer
- cancer du poumon = lung cancer
- cancer du rein = renal cancer
- cancer du sein = breast cancer

cancéreux *m*, **cancéreuse** *f* cancer patient
cancéreux,-euse *adj* cancerous; malignant
cancérigène *m*; **cancérogène** *m*; **also** *adj* carcinogen; cancer-causing; carcinogenic
cancérologue *m,f* cancer specialist
Candida albicans Candida albicans (a fungus)
candidose *f* **(syn. moniliase)** thrush; candidosis; candidiasis; moniliasis
canine *f* canine (tooth), eye tooth
cannabis *m* cannabis
canne *f* walking stick; cane
- canne anglaise = (forearm) crutch
- canne avec quadripode = quadruped stick
- canne blanche = white stick

capacité *f* capacity
capsule *f* capsule
carabin *m* **(students' slang)** medical student
carbone *m*, **oxyde de; carbone, monoxyde de** carbon monoxide
carcinogène *m*; **also** *adj* carcinogen
carcinome *m* carcinoma
cardiaque *adj* cardiac
- être cardiaque = to suffer/ to have a heart condition
- je suis cardiaque = I have heart trouble

cardio-vasculaire *adj* cardiovascular
cardiogramme *m* cardiogram
cardiographe *m* cardiograph
cardiographie *f* cardiography
cardiologie *f* cardiology
cardiologue *m,f* cardiologist
cardite *f* carditis
carence *f* deficiency
- carence vitaminique; carence en vitamines = vitamin deficiency
- maladie de/par carence = deficiency disease

carie *f* caries
- carie dentaire = dental caries; tooth decay
- j'ai une carie = I have got a bad tooth

21

carnet *m* **de santé** health record
carnet *m* **de vaccination** vaccination record
caroncule *f* **lacrymale** lachrymal caruncle, lachrymal duct
carotène *m* carotene
carotide *f* [AM: artères corotides du cou et de la tête] carotid [AM: carotid arteries of the neck and head]
carotidien *adj* carotid
carpe *m* carpus, carpal
carpes *mpl* [AM: les os du poignet] carpals [AM: wrist bones]
carte *f* **vitale** medical registration card (France)
cartilage *m* cartilage
cas *m* case
casque *m* **de sécurité** safety helmet; hard hat
casser *v* to break
  ▪ cassé = broken
  ▪ se casser une côte = to break one's rib
castration *f* castration
catalepsie *f* catalepsy; trance
  ▪ tomber en catalepsie = to fall or go into a trance
cataplasme *m* poultice; cataplasm
  ▪ cataplasme de farine de lin = linseed meal poultice
  ▪ cataplasme de moutarde = mustard poultice
  ▪ cataplasme sinapisé = mustard poultice; mustard plaster
cataracte *f* cataract
  ▪ il a été opéré de la cataracte = he has been operated on for a cataract
catarrhal,-e *adj* catarrhal
catarrhe *m* catarrh
catgut *m* catgut
cathartique *m*; also *adj* cathartic
cathéter *m* catheter
cathétérisme *m* catheterization
cauchmar *m* nightmare
cautérisation *f* cauterization
caverneux,-euse *adj* cavernous; hollow
  ▪ poumon caverneux = lung with cavitations; lung with cavernous lesion
cavité *f* cavity
  ▪ cavité abdominale = abdominal cavity
  ▪ cavité articulaire = socket (of bone)
  ▪ cavité buccale = oral cavity
  ▪ cavité nasale = nasal cavity
  ▪ cavité pleurale = pleural cavity

- cavité pulpaire = pulp cavity (tooth)

cécité *f* blindness

ceinture *f* **herniaire** truss

ceinture *f* **orthopédique** surgical corset

cellule *f* cell

- cellule sanguine = blood cell

cellulite *f* 1 cellulitis; 2 cellulite

centre *m* **anti-poison** poison centre

centre *m* **de convalescence** convalescent home

centre *m* **sanitaire** health care centre

céphalée *f*; **céphalalgie** *f* headache

- céphalée de tension = tension headache

céphalo-rachidien,-ienne *adj* cerebrospinal

- liquide céphalo-rachidien = cerebrospinal fluid

cérébral,-e *adj* cerebral

cérébro-spinal,-e *adj* cerebrospinal

cerne *m* **(autour des yeux)** ring (under the eye)

certificat *m* **de vaccination** vaccination certificate

certificat *m* **médical** medical certificate

cérumen *m* cerumen; earwax

cerveau *m* cerebrum; brain

cervelet *m* cerebellum

césarienne *f* [AM: incision permettant d'extraire un nouveau-né de l'utérus] Caesarean (section) [AM: incision allowing delivery of baby from the uterus]

- elle a eu une césarienne = she had a Caesarean

chalazion *m* [AM: petite nodule dans la paupière] chalazion [AM: small cyst in or on eyelid]

chambre *f* **de travail préparatoire à l'acouchement** labour room

champ *m* **visuel; champ** *m* **de vision** field of vision; visual field

champignon *m* fungus; mushroom

- champignon hallucinogène = hallucinogenic mushroom; magic mushroom
- champignon vénéneux = poisonous toadstool

chancre m chancre

- chancre mou; chancrelle *f* = chancroid; soft chancre
- chancre syphilitique = chancre

charbon *m* anthrax

charbon *m* **activé** activated charcoal; activated carbon

chauffe-biberon *m* bottle warmer (baby's bottle)

chauve *adj* bald

chef *m* **de service** medical consultant

cheveux *mpl* hair (head)

- chute des cheveux = loss of hair

23

cheville *f* ankle
- je me suis tordu la cheville = I have twisted my ankle

chimiotherapie *f* chemotherapy

chiropracteur *m* chiropractor

chiropractie *f*; **chiropraxie** *f* chiropractic

chirurgie *f* surgery

chirurgie *f* **cardiaque** heart surgery

chirurgie *f* **maxillaire** jaw surgery

chirurgie *f* **ophtalmique** eye surgery

chirurgie *f* **plastique** plastic surgery

chirurgien *m*, **chirurgienne** *f* surgeon

chirurgien *m* **cardiaque; chirurgienne** *f* **cardiaque; cardiochirurgien(ne)** *m(f)* heart surgeon

chirurgien *m* **plastique; chirurgienne** *f* **plastique** plastic surgeon

Chlamydiae *f* Chlamydiae

choc *m* shock
- choc anaphylactique = anaphylactic shock
- choc cardiogénique = cardiac shock
- choc électrique = electric shock
- choc nerveux = (nervous) shock
- choc opératoire = post-operative shock
- elle est sous le coup de choc = she is suffering from shock
- en état de choc = in a state of shock
- état de choc = state of shock

choléra *m* cholera

cholestérol *m* cholesterol

choquer *v* to shake; to shock
- être choqué = to be in shock

chorée *f* chorea; St. Vitus' dance
- chorée de Huntingdon = Huntingdon's chorea

choroïde *f* [AM: membrane du globe oculaire] choroid [AM: eyeball membrane]

choroidite *f* [AM: inflammation de la choroide] choroiditis [AM: inflammation of the choroid]

chromosome *m* chromosome
- chromosome X ou Y = X or Y chromosome

chronique *adj* chronic

chute *f* **des reins** small of the back

chyle *m* chyle

cicatrice *f* scar
- tissus mpl cicatrisés = scar tissue

cicatrisant,-e *adj* healing
- cicatrisant m = healing product

24

cicatrisation *f* healing
cicatriser *v* to heal
- ça devrait cicatriser rapidement = it should heal quickly
cil *m* eyelash
circoncision *f* circumcision
circulation *f* circulation
- circulation sanguine = circulation of blood
cire *f* wax
- applicateur de cire = wax applicator
- cire d'abeilles = beeswax
- épilation à la cire = waxing (hair removal)
cirrhose *f* cirrhosis
- cirrhose du foie = cirrhosis of the liver
ciseaux *mpl* scissors
ciseaux *mpl* **à ongles** nail scissors
civière *f* stretcher; hospital trolley
claustrophobie *f* claustrophobia
clavicule *f* clavicle; collarbone
clinique *f* 1 clinic (hospital department); 2 nursing home; private clinic
- clinique d'accouchement = maternity home
- clinique prénatale = prenatal cliniic
clitoris *m* clitoris
cloison *f* **(du nez)** septum (of nose)
clone *m* clone
cloner *v* to clone
cloquer *v* to blister
- cloqué = blistered
clou *m* boil; furuncle
coagulant *m* coagulant
coagulation *f* coagulation
cocaïne *f* cocaine
coccyx *m* coccyx
cochléaire *adj* cochlear
cochlée *f* **(syn. limaçon osseux)** [AM: cavité enroulé en spirale de l'oreille interne]
    cochlea [AM: spiral cavity of internal ear]
code *m* **génétique** genetic code
codéine *f* codeine
cœur *m* heart
- j'ai le coeur malade = I have a heart condition
- opération à cœur ouvert = open-heart surgery
col *m* neck

- col de la vessie = neck of the bladder
- col de l'utérus; col utérin = cervix of uterus; neck of the womb
- col du fémur = neck of the thigh bone

colère *f* 1 anger; 2 fit; tantrum
colibacille *m* *Escherichia coli*
colibacillose *f* colibacillosis
colique *f* diarrhoea; colic
- colique biliare = biliary colic
- colique hépatique = biliary colic, hepatic colic
- colique néphrétique = renal colic; nephritic colic
- coliques = gripe; gripes
- coliques de plomb = lead poisoning colic
- j'ai les coliques = I have diarrhoea; stomach pain; colic pain; colic

colite *f* [AM: inflammation du colon] colitis [AM: inflammation of the colon]
collagène *m*; **also adj** collagen
collutoire *m* oral medication; throat spray (in atomiser can)
collyre *m* eye wash; eye lotion
côlon *m* colon
- côlon irritable = irritable colon

colonne *f* **vertébrale (syn. colonne rachidienne; rachis)** vertebral column; spinal column
colopathie *f* **fonctionnelle** irritable bowel syndrome
coloration *f* tinting (hair)
- produit *m* de coloration = tinting/colouring product for hair

coloscopie *f* [AM: examen visuel de l'intérieur du côlon] coloscopy [AM: visual examination of interior of colon]
coma *m* coma
- dans un coma dépassé = brain-dead
- être/entrer dans le coma = to be/ to go into a coma

comédon *m* blackhead; comedo
commotion *f* concussion; shock
- commotion cérébrale = concussion
- commotion électrique = electric shock
- commotion mentale = mental shock

commotionner *v* **(quelqu'un)** to give (someone) a shock
- commotionné = in a state of shock; suffering from concussion
- être fortement commotionné = to be severely shocked
- une décharge électrique l'a commotionné = he has received a severe electric shock

communiquer *v* **(une maladie)** to pass on (an illness)
compatibilité *f* **sanguine** blood compatibility

compère-loriot *m* (nom pop. de l'orgelet) sty(e)
complément *m* **alimentaire** food supplement
complications *fpl* complications
compresse *f* compress
compresse *f* **désinfectante** antiseptic compress
compresse *f* **stérilisée** sterilized dressing
compresser *v* to compress
compressif,-ive *adj* compressive
comprimé *m* tablet
- comprimé d'aspirine = aspirin tablet
- comprimé de vitamine = vitamin tablet
- comprimé pelliculé = coated tablet
- comprimé sublingual (linguette) = under-tongue tablet
- prenez les comprimés avant/après les repas = take the tablets before/after meals
- prenez les comprimés avec un verre d'eau = take the tablets with water
- prenez les comprimés le matin/le soir = take the tablets in the morning/at night
compte-gouttes *m* dropper
conception *f* conception
concrétion *f* concretion (eg of a calculus)
condamner *v* to give up (hope for)
- condamné = terminal
conditionneur *m* conditioner
conduits *mpl* **lacrymaux** lachrymatory ducts
congé *m* **de maladie** sick leave
congénital,-e *adj* congenital
congestion *f* congestion
- congestion cérébrale = stroke (cerebrovascular accident)
- congestion pulmonaire = congestion of the lungs
conjonctive *f* [AM: membrane de la paupière] conjunctiva [AM: membrane of the eyelid]
conjonctivite *f* [AM: inflammation de la conjonctive] conjunctivitis [AM: inflammation of the conjunctiva]
connaissance f consciousness
- il est resté sans connaissance pendant une heure = he remained unconscious for an hour
- perdre connaissance = to become unconscious
- tomber sans connaissance = to faint
consanguinité *f* consanguinity
conscience *f* 1 awareness; 2 consciousness; 3 conscience
- perdre/reprendre conscience = to lose/regain consciousness
conseiller *v* to advise; to recommend

cordon

consolider v (une fracture) to set (a fracture)
constipation f constipation
constipé,-e adj constipated
constiper v to constipate; to make constipated
- constipé = constipated
- constipé, constipée (m,f) = person suffering constipation
constitution f constitution
consultation f consultation
- aller à la consultation = to visit the surgery; to visit the doctor's office
- service (hospitalier) de consultation externe = outpatients' clinic
contact m contact
- ça s'attrape par le contact = it's contagious
contagion f contagion; contagiousness
contaminer v to contaminate
- contaminé = contaminated
contention f support (eg bandage, splint, plaster, brace); setting
contraceptif m contraceptive
contraception f contraception
contraction f contraction
contractions utérines = uterine contractions
contracture f [AM: contraction involontaire prolongée des muscles, par ex. crampe]
contracture [AM: involuntary prolonged muscular contraction, eg cramp]
contre-indication f contraindication
- les contra-indications d'un médicament = the contraindications of a medicine
contrepoison m antidote
contrôle m des naissances (syn. planification familiale) birth control; family planning
contusion f bruise
contusionner v to bruise
- un bras/un genou contusionné = a bruised arm/knee
convalescence f convalescence
convulsion f convulsion
coqueluche f whooping cough
cor m corn (on foot)
- cor emplâtre = corn plaster (protector)
- pansement pour le cor = corn remover/softener plaster
corde f spinale (syn. moelle épinière) spinal cord
corde f vocale vocal cord
cordon m cord
- cordon médullaire = spinal cord
- cordon ombilical = umbilical cord

- cordon spermatique = spermatic cord
- cordons de la moelle épinière = medullary cords

cornée *f* cornea (eye)

coronaire *adj* coronary

corps *m* body
- corps étranger = foreign body
- corps jaune = yellow body, corpus luteum
- corps vitré = vitreous body (eye)
- le corps médical = the medical profession

corpulence *f* corpulence; stoutness
- de faible/forte/moyenne corpulence = of slight/stout/medium build

corriger *v* to correct (eg vision)

corrompre *v* to contaminate (eg blood)

cortex *m* cortex
- le cortex cérébral = the cerebral cortex

cortisone *f* cortisone

coryza *m* cold in the head; coryza; rhinitis

côte *f* rib

coton *m* cotton wool
- coton démaquillant = make-up remover pad
- coton hydrophile = cotton wool; absorbent cotton
- coton-tige ® *m* = cotton-bud; cotton applicator

cou *m* neck

cou-de-pied *m* instep

couche *f* **pour bébés** nappy; diaper
- couche en cellulose = disposable nappy/diaper
- couche jetable = disposable nappy/diaper

couche *f* **pour incontinents** incontinence pad

couche-culotte *f* nappy (baby's); diaper (disposable)

couches *fpl* confinement ; childbirth
- elle a eu des couches pénibles = she had a difficult labour
- fausse couche = miscarriage
- mourir en couches = to die in childbirth
- retour de couches = resumption of menses (after childbirth)
- une femme en couches = a woman in labour

coude *m* elbow

couenne *f* **inflammatoire** buffy coat

coup *m* **de chaleur** heatstroke

coup *m* **de froid** chill

coup *m* **de pompe** breakdown; exhaustion

coup *m* **de soleil** sunburn; slight sunstroke

crépitation

coupe-faim *m* appetite suppressant
coupe-ongles *m* nail clippers
couperose *f* (syn: acné rosacée) acne rosacea
coupure *f* cut
courbatures *fpl* aches and pains; weakness
  ▪ avoir des courbatures = to be stiff
  ▪ j'ai des courbatures = I am feeling weak; I have aches and pains
couronne *f* crown (of tooth)
  ▪ couronne dentaire = dental crown; capping
couveuse *f* incubator
crampe *f* cramp
  ▪ crampes d'estomac = stomach cramps
  ▪ crampes musculaires = muscular cramps
  ▪ j'ai des crampes = I am having cramp(s)
  ▪ j'ai une crampe à la jambe = I have a cramp in my leg
crampe *f* **de poitrine** angina pectoris
crâne *m* cranium; skull
crayon *m* **à lèvres** lip liner; lip pencil
crayon *m* **à sourcils** eyebrow pencil
crayon *m* **de maquillage** make-up pencil
crayon *m* **pour les yeux** eyeliner
crème *f* cream
  ▪ crème à épiler = hair remover cream
  ▪ crème à raser = shaving cream
  ▪ crème antirides = anti-wrinkle cream
  ▪ crème antirougeurs = cream for red skin/ erythema cream
  ▪ crème antiseptique = antiseptic cream
  ▪ crème contre les insectes = insect repellant
  ▪ crème contre les rougeurs = nappy rash cream
  ▪ crème de base = foundation cream
  ▪ crème de jour = day cream
  ▪ crème démaquillante = cleansing cream
  ▪ crème dépilatoire = hair removing cream
  ▪ crème hydratante = moisturizing cream; moisturiser
  ▪ crème pour bébés = baby's cream
  ▪ crème pour le visage = face cream
  ▪ crème pour les mains = hand cream
  ▪ crème solaire = suntan lotion
  ▪ crème solaire facteur 8 = suntan lotion factor 8
crépitation *f* crepitation; crackling
  ▪ crépitation articulaire = articulary crepitation

- crépitation osseuse = bony crepitation; crepitus
- crépitation pulmonaire = crepitations

crétinisme *m*   cretinism

Creutzfeldt-Jakob, maladie de   Creutzfeldt-Jakob disease

crevasser *v*   to chap (eg skin)
- se crevasser = to become chapped

crise *f*   attack; fit; crisis
- crise cardiaque = heart attack
- crise d'appendicite = appendicitis
- crise d'asthme = asthma attack
- crise d'épilepsie = epileptic fit
- crise de foie = bilious or liverish attack
- crise de toux = coughing attack/fit
- piquer/faire une crise = to throw a tantrum; to throw a fit

Crohn, maladie de (syn: iléite régionale) [AM: inflammation chronique de l'iléon terminal]   Crohn's disease [AM: chronic enteritis affecting terminal part of ileum]

croissance *f*   growth (eg of a child)

croup *m*   croup

croûte *f*   scab

cubitus *m*   [AM: os interne de l'avant-bras]   ulna [AM: inner bone of forearm]

cuillerée *f* **à café**   teaspoonful (eg of medicine)
- prenez deux cuillerées après les repas = take two teaspoonsfuls after meals.

cuillerée *f* **à soupe**   tablespoonful

cuir *m* **chevelu**   scalp

cuisine *f* **minceur**   low-calorie dishes

cuisse *f*   thigh

curare *m*   curare

cure-dents *m*   toothpick

curetage *m*; **curettage** *m*   curettage

curette *f*   curette; scraper

Cushing, syndrome de [AM: syndrome causé par l'hyperproduction de glucocorticoïdes]   Cushing's syndrome [AM: syndrome due to the overproduction of glucocorticoids]
- maladie de Cushing = Cushing's disease

cyanose *f*   cyanosis

cyclisme *m*   cycling
- faire beaucoup de vélo = to do a lot of cycling

cystite *f* [AM: inflammation de la vessie]   cystitis [AM: inflammation of the bladder]

D

daltonien *m*; **daltonienne** *f*; also *adj*   colour-blind person; colour-blind
daltonisme *m*   colour blindness; daltonism
danse *f*   dance
 ▪ avoir la danse de Saint-Guy = to have St Vitus's dance
débander *v*   to unbandage
débilité *f* **mentale**   mental deficiency
déboîtement *m* **(nom courant pour luxation)**   dislocation
déboîter *v*   to dislocate
 ▪ se déboîter le genou = to dislocate one's knee
décharge *f* **électrique (voir choc)**   electric shock
décharge *f*   discharge (of patient)
déchirer (se)   to tear (eg a muscle)
 ▪ se déchirer un muscle = to tear a muscle
déchirure *f*   tear; laceration
 ▪ déchirure abdominale/intercostale/musculaire = abdominal/intercostal/ muscle
 tear
décibel *m* **(dB)**   [AM: unité de mesure de l'intensité sonore]   decibel (dB)   [AM: unit of sound
intensity]
décollement *m*   detachment (eg of retina)
 ▪ décollement de la rétine = detachment of the retina
décoller (se) *v*   to become detached (eg retina)
décongestif *m*; **décongestif,-ive** *adj*   decongestant
décongestionnant *m*   decongestant
décongestionner *v*   to decongest; to relieve congestion in
défécation *f*   defecation
defenses *fpl* **immunitaires**   immune system
défibrillateur m   defibrillator
défibrillation f   defibrillation
défibriller *v*   to defibrillate
déficience *f*   deficiency
 ▪ déficience immunologique = immunodeficiency
 ▪ déficience intellectuelle = mental retardation
 ▪ déficience mentale = mental deficiency
 ▪ déficience musculaire = muscular insufficiency
déficient *m*; **déficient,-e** *adj*   deficient person; deficient *(adj)*
 ▪ enfant déficient = mentally deficient child; child with physical disability
 ▪ déficient mental/visuel = mentally/visually handicapped person
déformation *f*   deformation
dégagement *m*   delivery; expulsion; freeing (of baby in childbirth)

dégager *v* to clear (eg throat, nose, chest)
dégénération *f* degeneration
dégénéré *m*; **dégénérée** *f*; **also** *adj* medically degenerate person; degenerate
dégénérescence *f* degeneration; deterioration
  ▪ dégénérescence maculaire (DMLA) = macular degeneration
dégénérescent,-e *adj* degenerating; deteriorating
déglutir *v* to swallow
déglutition *f* act of swallowing; deglutition
degré *m* degree
  ▪ brûlure du premier/deuxième degré = first/second degree burn
  ▪ degré centigrade/Fahrenheit/Baumé = degree centigrade /Fahrenheit /Baumé
  ▪ degré de brûlure = degree of burns
déjection *f* evacuation; defecation
  ▪ déjections = faeces; excrement
délire *m* delirium
  ▪ délire de persécution = persecution mania
  ▪ délire hallucinatoire = hallucinatory delirium
délirer *v* to be delirious
delirium tremens delirium tremens
deltoïde *m*; **deltoïde** *adj* deltoid (muscle); deltoidal
démangeaison *f* **(voir aussi 'prurit')** itch; itching
  ▪ avoir des démangeaisons = to be itching
  ▪ j'ai des démangeaisons dans le dos/dans le pied = my back/foot is itching
démanger *v* to itch
  ▪ ça me démange au bras = my arm is itching
  ▪ le dos me démange = my back is itching
démaquillant *m* make-up remover
démêlant,-e *adj* detangling; untangling (hair)
  ▪ baume démêlant = detangling preparation/balm
démêloir *m* wide-toothed comb
démence *f* dementia; madness
  ▪ démence précoce = dementia praecox
dément *m*; **démente** *f*; **also** *adj* demented person; demented *(adj)*
démission *f* discharge (of patient)
dengue *f* dengue (fever); breakbone fever
dent *f*; **dents** *fpl* tooth, teeth
  ▪ dent creuse = hollow tooth
  ▪ dent de lait = milk tooth; baby tooth
  ▪ dent de sagesse = wisdom tooth
  ▪ dent gâtée = bad tooth
  ▪ dents artificiels = artificial teeth

déplacer

- dents de derrière; dents du fond = back teeth
- dents de devant = front teeth
- dents du bas = lower teeth
- dents du haut = upper teeth
- se brosser les dents = to brush one's teeth

dentaire *adj* dental
- carie dentaire = tooth decay

dental,-e *adj* dental

dentier *m* 1 dentures (prosthesis); 2 dental plate; 3 dentition (natural teeth)
- mon dentier est cassé = my dentures are broken
- vous pouvez le réparer? = can you repair them?

dentifrice *m*; **also** *adj* toothpaste; dentifrice
- dentifrice fluoré = fluoride toothpaste
- pâte dentifrice = toothpaste
- poudre dentifrice = tooth powder

dentine *f* dentine

dentiste *m/f* dentist
- j'ai besoin de voir un dentiste = I need to see a dentist
- s'aller chez le dentiste = to go to the dentist
- un rendez-vous chez le dentiste = a dental appointment

dentisterie *f* dentistry

dentition *f* teeth; dentition; teething

denture *f* 1 dentition; 2 set of teeth

dénuder *v* bare (to); strip (to)
- se dénuder = to strip off

déodorant *m* deodorant; antiperspirant
- déodorant en spray = spray-on deodorant
- déodorant en stick = stick deodorant

département *m* **d'oto-rhino-laryngologie** ear, nose and throat department

dépasser *v* to pass; to exceed
- ne pas dépasser la dose prescrite = do not exceed the prescribed dose

dépendance *f* addiction (to a drug)

dépilatoire *m* depilatory

dépiler *v* to cause hair loss; to remove hair from

dépistage *m* screening
- dépistage précoce = early detection; early screening
- dépistage systématique pour sida = mass screening for Aids

dépister *v* to detect (eg a disease)

déplacer *v* to displace (eg a joint)
- se déplacer une articulation = to put a joint out; to displace a joint
- se déplacer une vertèbre = to slip a disc

déplâtrage *m* removing plaster
- le déplâtrage d'un membre = taking a limb out of plaster/its plaster cast

déplâtrer *v* to take out of plaster

dépôt *m* deposit

dépression *f* depression
- dépression légère/modérée = slight/moderate depresssion
- dépression nerveuse = nervous breakdown
- dépression névrotique = neurotic depression
- dépression opératoire = post-operative depression

dermatite *f*, **dermite** *f* [AM: affection cutanée] dermatitis [AM: skin affection]

dermatologie *f* dermatology

dermatologiste *m,f* dermatologiste

descente *f* descent
- descente d'organe = prolapse of an organ

désensibilisation *f* desensitization

désensibiliser *v* to desensitize

déshydratation *f* dehydration

déshydraté,-e *adj* dehydrated

désinfectant *m*; **désinfectant,-e** *adj* disinfectant
- produit m désinfectant = disinfectant

désinfecter *v* to disinfect

désinfection *f* disinfection

désintoxication *f* detoxification

désintoxiquer *v* to detoxify

désordre *m* disorder
- désordre fonctionnel/hépatique = functional/liver disorder

désorientation *f* disorientation

détente *f* relaxation
- une demi-heure de détente = a half-hour of relaxation

détresse *f* **respiratoire** respiratory distress syndrome; respiratory difficulties

déviation *f* deviation; inversion (of an organ); displacement (of uterus); curvature (of spine)
- déviation de la colonne vertébrale = curvature of the spine

dextrose *m* dextrose

diabète *m* diabetes
- diabète insipide = diabetes insipidus
- diabète latent = latent diabetes
- diabète sucré = diabetes mellitus
- être diabétique = to have diabetes; to be diabetic
- faire diabète = to have diabetes; to suffer from diabetes

diabétique *adj* diabetic

- je suis diabétique = I am diabetic
diagnose *f* diagnosis
diagnostic *m* diagnosis
diagnostique *adj* diagnostic
diagnostiquer *v* to diagnose
dialyse *f* **rénale** renal dialysis
dialyseur *m* dialyser
diaphragme *m* diaphragm
diarrhée *f* diarrhoea
- diarrhée des voyageurs = travellers' diarrhoea
- j'ai la diarrhée = I've got diarrhoea
diète *f* diet
diététicien *m*; **diététicienne** *f* dietician
diétiste *m* dietician; dietist
difformité *f* abnormality
difformité *f* **(congénitale)** deformity (congenital)
- présenter des difformités = to be deformed
digérer *v* to digest
digestibilité *f* digestibility
digestible *adj* digestible
digestif,-ive *adj* digestive
digestion *f* digestion
digitaline *f* digitalis
dilatateur *m*; **also** *adj* dilator; dilatator
dilatation *f* dilation; dilatation
- dilatation de la pupille = dilation of the pupil
diphtérie *f* diphtheria
diplégie *f* diplegia
discal,-e *adj* of an invertebratal disc
- hernie discale = slipped disc
dislocation *f* dislocation
disloquer *v* to dislocate
- disloqué,-e *adj* = dislocated
- se disloquer l'épaule = to dislocate one's shoulder
disque *m* disc
- disque intervertébral = intervertebral disc
dissolvant *m* nail varnish remover; solvent
distome *m* **(syn. douve)** fluke
diurétique *m*; **also** *adj* diuretic
diverticule *m* diverticulum
diverticulite *f* [AM: inflammation des diverticules du côlon] diverticulitis [AM: inflammation

of diverticula of the colon]

docteur *m* doctor
- docteur en médecine = doctor of medicine

doightier *m* fingerstall

doigt *m* finger
- doigt de pied = toe
- doigt en marteau = mallet finger
- petit doigt = little finger

don *m* **d'organes** donation of organs

don *m* **du sang** blood donation

donneur *m*; **donneuse** *f* donor
- donneur de sang = blood donor

dopamine *f* dopamine

dorsal,-e *adj* dorsal

dos *m* back
- j'ai mal dans le dos = I have pain in my back
- mal de dos = backache

dosage *m* amount; proportion; quantity determination; dosage (eg of medicine)

dose *f* dose (eg of medicine)

doser *v* measure (to); measure out (to)

dossier *m* **médical** medical dossier

douche *f* **vaginale** douche

douleur *f* ache; pain
- quelle genre de douleur éprouver vous? = what kind of pain is it ?
- une douleur aiguë = a sharp pain
- une douleur intermittente = an intermittent pain
- une douleur irritante = a nagging pain
- une douleur lancinante = a throbbing pain
- une douleur persistante = a constant pain
- une douleur sourde = a dull ache

douloureux,-euse *adj* painful; aching

douve *f* **(nom courant du 'distome')** fluke

Down, syndrome de Down's syndrome; mongolism

dragée *f* sugar-coated pill

drain *m* drain; drainage tube

drainage *m* drainage
- drainage lymphatique = lymphatic drainage

drainer *v* drain (to)

drip *m* **feeding** drip feeding

drip *m* **transfusion** drip transfusion

drogue *f* drug

- drogue dure/ douce = hard/soft drug

drogué *m*; **droguée** *f* drug addict

droguer *v* to dose up; to give drugs to
- se droguer = to take drugs; to be on drugs

droit *m* **médical** medical law

duodénite *f* [AM: inflammation du duodénum] duodenitis [AM: inflammation of the duodenum]

duodénum *m* [AM: partie de l'intestin] duodenum [AM: part of the intestine]

durée *f* **de l'hospitalisation** duration of hospitalisation

durillon *m* callus

dysenterie *f* dysentery

dysfonction *f*; **dysfonctionnement** *m* dysfunction

dyslexie *f* dyslexia

dyslexique *m,f*; **also** *adj* dyslexic person

dysménorrhée *f* dysmenorrhoea

dyspepsie *f* dyspepsia

dysphasie *f* dysphasia

dystrophie *f* [AM: nutrition déficiente entraînant dégénérescence du tissu] dystrophy [AM: defective nutrition leading to wasting of tissue]
- dystrophie musculaire = muscular dystrophy

dysurie *f* [AM: difficulté à uriner] dysuria [AM: difficulty in urinating]

E

eau *f*; **eaux** *fpl* water
- elle a perdu les eaux = her waters have broken

eau *f* **de Cologne** eau de Cologne

eau *f* **de Javel** bleach, household (liquid)

eau *f* **de parfum** eau de parfum

eau *f* **de toilette** eau de toilette

eau *f* **dentifrice** mouthwash

eau *f* **oxygénée** hydrogen peroxide

éblouissement *m* 1 dazzle; 2 dizzy spell
- avoir un éblouissement (étourdissement) = to have a dizzy turn/spell

ébouillanter *v* to scald
- s'ébouillanter = to scald oneself
- s'ébouillanter la main = to scald one's hand

écarteur *m* retractor

ecchymose *f* bruise
écharde *f* splinter
écharpe *f* sling (bandage)
- en écharpe = in a sling
échauffement *m* 1 inflammation; 2 overheating; 3 gonorrhea (pop. term)
- échauffement du ventre = constipation
échauffer *v* to overheat
- échauffer la peau = to inflame the skin
- échauffer le sang = to overheat the blood
- je suis un peu échauffé = I'm a bit constipated
échocardiographie *m* echocardiography; ultrasound cardiography
échographe *m* ultrasound scanner
échographie *f* ultrasound scan
- passer une échographie = to have an ultrasonic scan
- se faire faire une échographie = to have an ultrasound scan
échographier *v* to scan ultrasonically
échographique *adj* ultrasonic
éclampsie *f* eclampsia
éclissage *m* splinting; fixing bones with screwed plates
éclisse *f* splint
éclisser *v* to put in splints
écorchure *f* abrasion
écouler *v* to seep; to ooze (out) (eg pus)
écran *m* **solaire** sunscreen (cosmet)
- crème écran total = sun block
eczéma *m* eczema
édulcorant *m* **de synthèse** artificial sweetener
effet m effect
- effets secondaires = side effects
efficacité *f* effectiveness; efficacy
- efficacité thérapeutique = therapeutic effectiveness
effleurage *m* effleurage; light massage
effleurer *v* to touch/massage lightly
élancement *m* shooting pain; sharp pain; twinge
électrocardiogramme *m* electrocardiogram
électrocardiographe *m* electrocardiograph
électrocardiographie *f*, **ECG** electrocardiography
électroencéphalogramme *m*; **EEG** [AM: trace graphique des rythmes électriques cérébraux] electroencephalogram; EEG [AM: graphical trace of electrical activity of the brain]
électroencéphalographe *m* electroencephalograph

électroencéphalographie *f*; **EEG**   electroencephalography
électrothérapie *f*   electrotherapy
élimination *f*   elimination
éliminer *v*   to eliminate
élongation *f*   1 strained or pulled muscle; 2 traction
  ▪ se faire une élongation au mollet = to strain or pull a calf muscle
émail *m*   enamel (tooth)
embarras *m*   upset
  ▪ embarras gastrique = upset stomach; stomach upset
embarrasser *v*   to hinder; to embarrass
  ▪ avoir l'estomac embarrassé = to have an upset stomach
  ▪ embarrasser l'estomac = to lie heavy on the stomach
  ▪ j'ai la langue embarrassée = my tongue is coated
embolie *f*   embolism
  ▪ embolie artérielle = arterial embolism
  ▪ embolie cérébrale = cerebral embolism
embrocation *f*   embrocation
embryologie *f*   embryology
embryon *m*   embryo
  ▪ embryon congelé = frozen embryo
embryonnaire *adj*   embryonic
émétique *m*   emetic
éminence *f*   protuberance
émollient *m*; **émollient,-ente** *adj*   demulcent; emollient
émotion *f*   emotion
emphysème *m*   emphysema
  ▪ emphysème pulmonaire = emphysema of the lungs
empirique *m*; **empirique** *adj*   empiric
  ▪ remède empirique = empirical remedy
emplâtre *m*   1 plaster; 2 sticking plaster
  ▪ emplâtre pour les cors = corn plaster
empoisonnement *m* **(syn. intoxication)**   poisoning
empoisonnement *m* **du sang**   blood poisoning
empoisonner *v*   to poison
émulsion *f*   emulsion
enceinte *adj*   pregnant
  ▪ depuis combien de temps êtes-vous enceinte? = since when have you been
    pregnant?
  ▪ être enceinte de jumeaux = to be pregnant with twins
  ▪ être enceinte de trois mois = to be three months pregnant
  ▪ je suis enceinte = I am pregnant

encéphale *m*   brain; encephalon

encéphalite *f* [AM: inflammation de l'encéphale]   encephalitis [AM: inflammation of the brain]

encéphalogramme *m*   encephalogram

endémique *adj*   endemic

endocarde *m*   endocardium (of heart)

endocardite *f* [AM: inflammation de l'endocarde]   endocarditis [AM: inflammation of the endocardium]

endocrinologie *f*   endocrinoloy

endogène *adj* [AM: qui est dû à des causes interne]   endogenous [AM: produced from within (the body)]

endomètre *m* [AM: muqueuse tapissant la face interne de l'utérus]   endometrium [AM: lining membrane of uterus]

endométrite *f* [AM: inflammation de la muqueuse utérine]   endometritis [AM: inflammation of the uterine lining]

endoscope *m* [AM: instrument permettant d'observer l'intérieur d'une cavité]   endoscope [AM: instrument for inspecting interior of a cavity]

endoscopie *f*   endoscopy

enfant *m,f*   child
- enfant bleu = blue baby

enfant *m* **mort-né;enfant** *f* **mort-née**   stillbirth

enfler *v*   to swell up; to swell
- mon genou a beaucoup enflé = my knee has swollen up a lot

enflure *f*   swelling

enfoncement *m*   crushing; breaking
- il souffre d'un enfoncement de la boîte crânienne = he has a fractured skull
- il souffre d'un enfoncement de la cage thoracique = he has crushed ribs

engelure *f*   chilblain
- j'ai une engelure à mon pied = I have a chilblain on my foot

engorgement *m*   engorgement; obstruction

engorger *v*   to engorge; to obstruct

engouement *m*   obstruction (eg of a cavity); choking up (of hernia)

engourdissement *m*   numbness

enlever *v*   to remove; to take out (eg organ)

enlèvement *m*   removal (eg of an organ)

entérite *f* [AM: inflammation de la muqueuse de l'intestin grêle]   enteritis [AM: inflammation of the lining of the small intestine]

entérobactérie *f*   enterobacteria

entérocolite *f*   enterocolitis

entérovirus *m*   enterovirus

entorse *f*   sprain
- se faire une entorse au poignet = to sprain one's wrist

41

enveloppement *m*   pack
- enveloppement froid = cold pack
- enveloppement glacé = ice-pack

enzyme *f* ou *m*   enzyme

épanchement *m*   effusion
- avoir un épanchement de synovie = to have water on the knee

épaule *f*   shoulder
- épaule bloquée = frozen shoulder

épicondylite *f*   epicondylitis; tennis elbow

épidémie *f*   epidemic

épiderme *m*   epidermis

épididyme *m*   epididymis

épiglotte f   epiglottis

épilation *f*   removal of unwanted hair; epilation
- épilation à la cire = waxing

épilatoire *m;* **also** *adj*   hair remover; hair-removing; depilatory

épilepsie *f*   epilepsy

épileptique *m,f*   epileptic

épileptique *adj*   epileptic
- crise *f* d'épilepsie = epileptic fit

épiler *v*   to remove unwanted hair

épingle *f* **de sûreté**   safety pin

épingle *f* **à cheveux**   hairpin

épistaxis *f* [AM: saignement de nez]   epistaxis [AM: nose bleeding]

épithélial,-e *adj*   epithelial
- tissu épithélial = epithelial tissue

épithélioma *m;* **épithéliome** *m* [AM: tumeur maligne d'un tissu épithélial]   epithelioma; carcinoma [AM: malignant tumour of epithelial tissue]

épithélium *m* [AM: tissu de revêtement qui recouvre les surfaces internes/externes]   epithelium [AM: membranous tissue covering most internal/external surfaces]

éponge *f*   sponge

épreuve *f*   test; trial

épreuve *f* **de tolérance au glucose**   glucose tolerance test

épuisement *m*   exhaustion
- épuisement dû à la chaleur = heat exhaustion

épuration *f*   purification

épuration *f* **extrarénale**   dialysis

éraflure *f*   graze; scratch
- s'erafler = to graze/scratch oneself

ergothérapie *f;* **thérapeutique** *f* **occupationnelle**   occupational therapy

ergothérapeute *m,f*   occupational therapist

érosion *f* **(syn. exulcération)** abrasion; erosion

erratique *adj* erratic

éruption *f* 1 rash; 2 eruption (of tooth)
- avoir une éruption = to come out in a rash
- éruption d'une dent = eruption of a tooth

érysipèle *m*; **érésipèle** *m* [AM: maladie streptococcique de la peau] erysipelas [AM: streptoccocal infection of the skin]

érythème *m* erythema

érythème m fessier nappy rash
- avoir les fesses irritées = to have nappy rash

érythrocyte *m* **(syn. globule rouge; hématie)** [AM: cellule sanguine rouge] erythrocyte [AM: red blood cell]

érythromycine *f* [AM: antibiotique] erythromycin [AM: antibiotic]

escarre *f* bedsore

espérance *f* **de vie** life expectancy

estomac *m* stomach

étanche *adj* waterproof

éternuement *m* sneeze; sneezing

éternuer *v* to sneeze

étouffement *m* 1 asphyxiation; 2 suffocation; 3 choking; 4 breathlessness
- avoir des étouffements = to have fits of breathlessness
- mourir d'étouffement = to die of suffocation
- sensation d'étouffement = feeling of suffocation or breathlessness

étourdissement *m* giddiness

étrier *m* stirrup

euthanasie *f* euthanasia

évacuation *f* evacuation

évacuer *v* to evacuate; to discharge

évanoui *adj* unconscious
- il s'est évanoui = he is unconscious

évanouir *v*; **s'évanouir** to faint

évanouissement *m* fainting fit; fainting spell; blackout

éventration *f* eventration; rupture

évoluer *v* to evolve; to develop
- la maladie évolue = the illness is running its (normal) course

évolutif,-ive *adj* progressive

évolution *f* development; evolution

examen *m* examination
- examen cardiaque = heart examination
- examen clinique = clinical examination
- examen complémentaire = complementary examination (eg blood analysis,

radiography)
- examen cytobactériologique =cytobacteriological examination (eg of urine)
- examen de la vue = sight test
- examen du sang = blood test
- examen fonctionel = physical examination
- examen médical = medical examination
- examen prénuptial = pre-marital examination
- examen radiographique = x-ray examination; radiography
- examen radiologique = radiological examination (eg by x-rays)

examiner *v* to examine
exciter *v* to excite; to stimulate (eg nerve, muscle)
excrétion *f* excretion
excroissance *f* excrescence; outgrowth
expectorant *m*; **also** *adj* expectorant
- **extenseur** *m*; **also** *adj* extensor (muscle)

extension *f* stretching (eg of muscle); extension; traction (eg of limb)
externe *adj* external; exterior
extraction *f* extraction
extraire *v* to extract; to pull out (eg tooth)

F

face *f* face
faciès *m* features; facies
facteur *m* factor
- facteur Rhésus = Rhesus or Rh factor

faible *adj* weak
faiblesse *f* **mentale** mental defiiency
fantasme *m* fantasy; delusion
fard *m* make-up
- fard à joues = blusher
- fard à paupières = eye-shadow

fatigue *f* fatigue
- syndrome de fatigue chronique = chronic fatigue syndrome

fatiguer *v* to make tired; to get tired; to tire
- elle a le cœur fatigué = she has a weak heart

fausse couche *f* miscarriage

44

- faire une fausse couche = to have a miscarriage

fausses dents *fpl* false teeth

fauteuil *m* **roulant; fauteuil à roulettes (pour malades)** wheelchair

fébrifuge *m; also adj* febrifuge; antipyretic

fécondation *f* fertilization
  - fécondation in vitro = in vitro fertilization

fécondité *f* fertility

fémoral *adj* femoral (eg artery, nerve)

fémur *m* [AM: os de la cuisse] femur [AM: thigh bone]

fer *m* iron

fers *mpl* **(voir forceps)** forceps

fertilité *f* fertility

fesse *f* buttock
  - les fesses = the buttocks; the bottom

fessier,-ière *adj* buttock; gluteal
  - muscles fessiers = gluteal muscles

feuille *f* **de soins** statement of treatment

feuille *f* **de température** temperature chart

fibrillation *f* fibrillation
  - fibrillation auriculaire = auricular fibrillation
  - fibrillation ventriculaire = ventricular fibrillation

fibrose *f* **kystique** cystic fibrosis

fièvre *f* fever
  - fièvre cérébrale = brain fever
  - fièvre de Lassa = Lassa fever
  - fièvre ganglionnaire; fièvre glandulaire = glandular fever
  - fièvre paludéenne (voir paludisme) = malaria
  - fièvre paratyphoïde = paratyphoid fever
  - fièvre perpérale = puerperal fever
  - il a beaucoup de fièvre = he has a high temperature
  - j'ai 38 de fièvre = my temperature is 38 degrees
  - j'ai de la fièvre = I have a fever/ a high temperature

fiévreux, fiévreuse *adj* feverish
  - je me sens fiévreux (homme)/ fiévreuse (femme) = I feel feverish

fil *m* **dentaire** dental floss

filet *m* **à cheveux** hair net

filiforme *adj* thready (eg pulse)

fistule *f* fistula

flacon *m* small bottle; phial; flask
  - flacon doseur = small bottle with dropper

flamber *v* to sterilize (in a flame)

45

flatulence *f* flatulence
flatuosité *f* flatus
- avoir des flatuosités = to have wind
fléchir *v* to flex
fléchisseur *m*; **also** *adj* flexor (muscle)
fluor *m* flourine
fluoration *f* fluoridation
fluorure *m* fluoride
flush *m* flush
flux *m* flow
- flux de sang = flow of blood
- flux menstruel = menstrual flow
fluxion *f* swelling; inflammation; congestion
- fluxion dentaire = swelling; gumboil
- fluxion de poitrine = pneumonia
fœtus *m* foetus
foie *m* liver
- abcès du foie = abcess of the liver
- cancer du foie = cancer of the liver
folie *f* madness; lunacy; insanity
follicule *f* follicle
folliculite *f* folliculitis
fonctionnement *m* working; functioning
fond *m* **de teint** foundation (cosmet)
fontanelle *f* [AM: espace membraneux, non ossifié du crâne de nouveau-né] fontanelle [AM: non-bony part of baby's head]
forceps *m* forceps; pair of forceps
fouler (se) *v* to sprain; to twist
- avoir la cheville foulé = to have a sprained ankle
- se fouler le poignet/la cheville = to twist or sprain one's wrist/ankle
foulure *f* sprain
fourmillement *m* formication; pins and needles
fourmis *fpl* **dans les mains/jambes (avoir des)** to have pins and needles in the hands/ legs
fracture *f* fracture
- fracture compliqué = compound fracture
- fracture du crâne = fractured skull; fracture of the skull
- fracture fermée = simple fracture; closed fracture
- fracture ouverte = compound fracture; open fracture
fracturer *v* to fracture
- il s'est fracturé la jambe = he fractured his leg

fraise *f* strawberry; strawberry mark
fréquence *f* **cardiaque** heartbeat rate; pulse rate
fréquence *f* **respiratoire** respiration frequency; breathing rate
frictions *fpl* **localisées** localised frictional massage
frisson *m* chill; shiver
  ▪ j'ai des frissons = I am shivery
frissonner *v* to shiver (eg with fever)
froissement *m* **(d'un muscle)** strain (muscular)
froisser (se) *v* to strain (eg a muscle)
front *m* forehead
frottis *m* smear
  ▪ frottis sanguin = blood smear
  ▪ se faire faire un frottis cervicovaginal = to have a cervical smear
fumigateur *m* fumigator
furoncle *m* boil; furuncle

G

gale *f* **(syn. scabies** *f***)** scabies; itch
ganglion *m* ganglion
  ▪ avoir des ganglions = to have swollen glands
  ▪ ganglion lymphatique = lymph node; lymph gland
gangrène *f* gangrene
gant *m* **de toilette** flannel; face-flannel
gants *mpl* **latex** latex gloves
garde-malade *m,f* home nurse
gargariser *v*; **se gargariser** *v* to gargle
gargarisme *m* 1 gargle; mouthwash; 2 gargling
  ▪ se faire un gargarisme = to gargle
garrot *m* tourniquet
gastrectomie *f* [AM: résection partielle ou totale de l'estomac] gastrectomy [AM: removal of part or whole of the stomach]
gastrique *adj* gastric
gastrite *f* [AM: inflammation de la muqueuse de l'estomac] gastritis [AM: inflammation of the stomach lining]
gastroentérite *f* [AM: inflammation des muqueuses de l'estomac et de l'intestin] gastro-enteritis [AM: inflammation of lining of stomach and the intestine]
gel *m* **coiffant** hair gel

gel *m* **douche**   shower gel
gelée *f* **royale**   royal jelly
gélule *f*   gelatin capsule
gelure *f*   frostbite
gencive *f*   gum (of teeth)
 ▪ gencives = gums
gène *m*   gene
généraliser *v*   to generalize
 ▪ cancer généralisé = general cancer
 ▪ infection généralisée = systemic infection
 ▪ se généraliser = to spread (eg disease)
génétique *f*, **also** *adj*   1 genetics; 2 genetic *adj*
génie *m* **génétique**   genetic engineering
génome *m*   genome
 ▪ génome humain = human genome
genou *m*   knee
 ▪ mon genou s'est déboîté = my knee is dislocated
genouillère *f* **(bandage ou plâtre)**   knee support (bandage or plaster)
gerçure *f*   crack; chapping
 ▪ avoir les mains pleines de gerçures = to have badly chapped hands
gériatrie *f*   geriatrics
gériatrique *adj*   geriatric
germe *m*   germ
germe *m* **de blé**   wheat germ
 ▪ huile de germe de blé = wheat germ oil
gérontologie *f*   gerontology
gestation *f*   gestation; pregnancy
gibbosité *f*   hump; gibbosity
gingivite *f* [AM: inflammation de la gencive]   gingivitis [AM: inflammation of the gums]
ginkgo biloba *m*   ginkgo biloba
ginkgolide *m*   ginkgo biloba extract
ginseng *m*   ginseng
glaire *f*   1 mucus; 2 phlegm; 3 albumen (of an egg)
 ▪ avoir des glaires = to have catarrh
 ▪ glaire cervicale = cervical mucus
glaireux,-euse *adj*   mucous
glande *f*   gland
 ▪ glande endocrine = endocrine gland
 ▪ glande pituitaire (syn. hypophyse) = pituitary gland
 ▪ glande sébacée = sebaceous gland
 ▪ glande sudoripare = sweat gland

- glande surrénale; surrénale *f* = adrenal gland; suprarenal gland
- glande thyroïde = thyroid gland
- glandes digestives = digestive glands
- glandes lacrymales = lachrymatory glands
- glandes mammaires = mammary glands
- glandes salivaires = salivary glands

glandulaire *adj* glandular
glaucome *m* glaucoma
globe *m* **oculaire** eyeball
globule *m* **rouge/blanc** red/white blood cell
globule *m* **sanguin** blood cell; blood corpuscle
glotte *f* glottis
glucose *m* glucose
gluten *m* gluten
glycérine *f* **(syn. glycérol** *m*) glycerine
goitre *m* goitre; goiter
gommage *m* scrub (cosmet)
- se faire faire un gommage du corps/de visage = to have a body/facial scrub

gomme *f* gum; gumma (pathological)
gonade *f* gonad
gonflement *m* swelling (eg eyelid, feet); distension (eg stomach)
gonfler *v* to swell up; to become puffy (face, eyelid)
gonorrhée *f* **(syn. blennorragie)** gonorrhea; gonococcal urethritis
gorge *f* throat
- j'ai mal à la gorge = I have a sore throat

gourme *f* **(syn. impétigo)** impetigo (eg in children)
goût *m* taste
goutte *f* gout
goutte *f* drop (of liquid)
- avoir la goutte au nez = to have a dripping or runny nose
- être nourri au goutte-à-goutte = to be drip-fed
- goutte-à-goutte = drip
- gouttes pour le nez = nose drops
- gouttes pour les oreilles = ear drops
- gouttes pour les yeux = eyedrops

gouttière *f* splint; gutter
- gouttière sagittale = sagittal suture
- gouttière vertébrale = vertebral groove

grain *m* grain; pellet; small pill
grain *m* **de beauté (syn. lentigo; lentigine)** mole; beauty spot
grand malade *m* severely ill patient

49

grave *adj* serious
- une blessure grave = a serious injury

gravelle *f* gravel

greffe *f* transplant; graft
- greffe de peau = skin graft
- greffe de rein = kidney transplant
- greffe d'organes = organ transplant

greffer *v* to transplant; to graft

grelotter *v* **(de)** to shiver (with) (eg cold, fever)

grésillement *m* sizzling; crackling (noise)

grippal,-e *adj* influenza; flu
- affection grippale = flu
- état grippal = flu

grippe *f* influenza; flu
- elle a la grippe = she has influenza
- faire grippe = to get or to go down with influenza
- vaccin contre la grippe = influenza vaccine

grippe *f* **asiatique** Asian flu

grippe *f* **espagnole** Spanish flu

grippe *f* **gastro-intestinale** gastric flu

grossesse *f* pregnancy
- grossesse extra-utérine = ectopic pregnancy
- grossesse nerveuse = phantom pregnancy
- test *m* de grossesse = pregnancy test

grosseur *f* lump (tumour)
- avoir un grosseur au sein = to have a lump in the breast

grossir *v* 1 to put on weight (to); 2 to increase

groupe *m* **sanguin** blood group; blood type
- mon groupe sanguin est (A, B, AB, O) = my blood group is (A, B, AB, O)

guérir *v* to cure (eg illness); to make better; to heal (eg a wound)

guérison *f* recovery (eg from illness); healing (eg of a fracture); cure

guérissable *adj* curable

gueule *f* **de bois** hangover

gustatif,-ive *adj* gustative; gustatory

gymnase *m* gymnasium

gymnaste *m,f* gymnast

gymnastique *f* gymnastics
- gymnastique aquatique = aquagym
- gymnastique corrective = physiotherapy exercises
- gymnastique rhythmique et sportive; GRS = eurythmics
- gymnastique suédoise = callisthenics

gynécologie *f* gynaecology; gynecology
gynécologiste *m,f* gynaecologist
gynécologue *m,f* gynaecologist

H

haleine *f* breath; breathing
 ▪ mauvaise haleine = bad breath
halitose *f* halitosis
hallucination *f* hallucination
halluciné *m*; **hallucinée** *f* hallucinated person
hallucinogène *adj* hallucinogenic
hanche *f* hip
 ▪ prothèse de la hanche = hip replacement
handicap *m* disability; handicap
handicapé *m*; **handicapée** *f* disabled person
handicapé,-e *adj* handicapped; disabled
hématie *f* **(syn. érythrocyte; globule rouge)** [AM: cellule sanguine rouge] red blood
 cell [AM: red blood cell]
hématologie *f* haematology ; hematology
hématologique *adj* haematological
hématologiste *m,f* haematologist
hématologue *m,f* haematologist
hématoma *m* bruise; haematoma
hémiplégie *f* [AM: paralysie affectant une moitié du corps] hemiplegia [AM: paralysis of one
 side of the body]
hémiplégique *m/f* hemiplegic ; person paralyzed on one side
hémiplégique *adj* hemiplegic ; paralyzed on one side
hémodialyse *f* haemodialysis; hemodialysis
hémoglobine *f* haemoglobin; hemoglobin
hémolyse *f* haemolysis
hémophile *m,f* haemophiliac
hémophile *adj* haemophilic
hémophilie *f* haemophilia
hémorragie *f* haemorrhage; bleeding
hémorragie *f* **externe** external bleeding
hémorragie *f* **interne** internal bleeding
hémorroïdes *fpl* haemorrhoids; hemorrhoids; piles

51

- j'ai des hémorroïdes = I have haemorrhoids/piles
hémorroïdaire *adj*　haemorrhoidal; with haemorrhoids
hémorroïdal,-e *adj*　haemorrhoidal
héparine *f*　heparin
hépatique *m,f*　person who suffers from a liver complaint
hépatique *adj*　hepatic
hépatite *f*　hepatitis
- hépatite A = hepatitis A
- hépatite B = hepatitis B
- hépatite C = hepatitis C
- hépatite virale = viral hepatitis
herbe *f* **médicinale**　medicinal herb
hérédité *f*　heredity
hernie *f*　hernia; rupture
- hernie discale = slipped disc
- hernie étranglée = strangulated hernia
- hernie inguinale = inguinal hernia
herpès *m*　herpes
- herpès buccal = cold sores; herpes simplex
- herpès circiné = ringworm
- herpès de la lèvre = cold sore; herpes labialis
- herpès génital = genital herpes
- herpès zoster = shingles
hétérosexualité *f*　heterosexuality
hétérosexuel *m*; **hétérosexuelle** *f*; also *adj*　heterosexual
hibernation *f* **artificielle**　induced hypothermia
hirsutisme *m*　hirsutism
histamine *f*　histamine
histologie *f*　histology
Hodgkin, maladie *f* **de** [AM: affection cancéreuse]　Hodgkin's disease [AM: cancerous condition]
holistique *adj*　holistic
homéopathie *f* [AM: méthode thérapeutique]　homeopathy [AM: therapeutic method]
homéopathique *adj*　homeopathic
- à doses homéopathiques = in small doses
homosexualité *f*　homosexuality
homosexuel *m*; **homosexuelle** *f*; also *adj*　homosexual
hôpital *m*　hospital
- hôpital de jour = out-patient clinic
- hôpital d'enfants = children's hospital
- hôpital d'isolement = isolation hospital

- hôpital général = general hospital
- il faut aller à l'hôpital = you must go to hospital
- où est l'hôpital? = where is the hospital?

hoquet *m* hiccup; hiccough
- avoir le hoquet = to have hiccups

hoqueter *v* to hiccup; to hiccough

honoraires *mpl* **de médecin** doctor's fee

honoraires *mpl* **médicaux** medical fees

hormone *f* hormone

houppe *f* **(à poudrer)** powder puff

houppette *f* **(à poudrer)** powder puff

huile *f* oil
- huile de foie de morue = cod liver oil
- huile de germe de blé = wheat germ oil
- huile de ricin = castor oil
- huile de tournesol = sunflower oil
- huile d'olive = olive oil
- huile d'onagre = evening primrose oil
- huile essentielle = essential oil

humérus *m* [AM: os unique du bras] humerus [AM: bone of the upper arm]

humeur *f* humour
- humeur aqueuse/vitreuse; vitrée de l'œil = aqueous/vitreous humour (of the eye)

hydratation *f* hydration; moisturizing (eg of skin)

hydrate *m* **de chloral** chloral hydrate

hydrocéphalie *f* hydrocephalus

hydrocortisone *f* hydrocortisone

hydrocution *f* immersion syncope

hydronéphrose *f* hydronephrosis

hydropisie *f* **(terme mod. 'anasarque')** [AM: œdème généralisé du tissu] dropsy [AM: general oedema of the tissues]

hydrothérapie *f* hydrotherapy

hygiène *f* hygiene

hygiène *f* **du travail** industrial hygiene

hygroma *m* **(syn. bursite)** bursitis

hymen *m* hymen

hyperactif,-ive *adj* hyperactive

hyper- (préfixe); excès ou augmentation hyper- (prefix); excess or increase

hyperactivité *f* hyperactivity

hyperglycémie *f* hyperglycaemia; hyperglycemia
- épreuve d'hyperglycémie *f* provoquée = glucose tolerance test

ileite

hyperhidrose *f* hyperhidrosis; excess perspiration
hyperparathyroïdie *f* hyperparathyroidism
hypertensif,-ive *adj* hypertensive
hypertension *f* hypertension; high blood pressure
  ▪ hypertension artérielle = high blood pressure
  ▪ hypertension intracrânienne = intracranial hypertension
  ▪ je souffre d'hypertension = I have high blood pressure
hyperthermie *f* hyperthermia
hypertrophie *f* hypertrophy
hyperventilation *f* hyperventilation
  ▪ être en hyperventilation = to hyperventilate
hypnose *f* hypnosis
hypnothérapie *f* hypnotherapy
hypnotique *m*; **also** *adj* hypnotic; sleep inducing (eg sleeping pill)
hypo- (préfixe); insuffisance; diminution hypo- (prefix); insufficiency; decrease
hypoallergénique *adj* hypoallergenic
hypocondriaque *m,f*; **also** *adj* hypochondriac
hypocondrie *f* hypochondria
hypoglycémie *f* hypoglycaemia
hypophyse *f* pituitary gland
hypotensif,-ive *adj* hypotensive
hypotension *f* artérielle low blood pressure
hypothalamus *m* hypothalamus
hypothermie *f* hypothermia
hypothyroïdie *f* hypothyroidism
hystérectomie *f* [AM: ablation de l'utérus] hysterectomy [AM: removal of uterus]
hystérie *f* hysteria
hystérographie *f* uterography
hystéroscope *m* hysteroscope
hystéroscopie *f* hysteroscopy
hystérique *m,f*; **also** *adj* hysteric; hysterical
hémorragique *adj* haemorrhagic

I

ictère *m* jaundice; icterus
idiotie *f* idiocy
iléite *f* [AM: inflammation de l'iléon] ileitis [AM: inflammation of the ileum]

54

iléite *f* **régionale**   Crohn's disease; regional enteritis
iléon *m*   [AM: partie terminale de l'intestin grêle]   ileum [AM: lower part of the small intestine]
iliaque *adj*   iliac
- os iliaque = hip bone

imagerie *f* **par résonance magnétique; I.R.M.**   nuclear magnetic resonance imaging
imbécile *m,f*; also *adj*   imbecile; imbecilic
imbécillité *f*   imbecility; idiocy
immunisation *f*   immunization
immunité *f*   immunity
impétigo *m*   impetigo
implant *m*   implant
incubation *f*   incubation
incurable *m,f*; also *adj*   incurable
index *m*   1 index finger; forefinger; 2 index
indication *f*   indication
- indication thérapeutique = remedial indication

indigestion *f*   indigestion
infantile *adj*   infantile; child's; children's
infarctus *m*   [AM: nécrose d'un tissu à la suite d'un apport de sang insuffisant]   infarction; infarct [AM: dead tissue due to failure of blood supply]
infarctus *m* **du myocarde**   heart attack; coronary thrombosis; myocardial infarction
- avoir un infarctus = to have a coronary; to have a heart attack

infecter *v*   to infect
- c'est infecté = it's infected
- s'infecter = to become infected; to become septic
- un pied/doigt infecté = a poisoned/infected foot/finger

infectieux,-ieuse *adj*   infectious
infection *f*   infection
- vous avez une infection = you've got an infection

infertilité *f*   infertility
infestation *f*   infestation
infester *v*   to infest
infiltration *f*   injection; seepage; infiltration
- se faire faire des infiltrations = to have injections

infirme *m,f*   invalid
infirmier *m*   nurse (male)
infirmière *f*   nurse (female)
infirmière *f* **diplômée**   registered nurse; nurse with diploma
infirmière *f* **en chef**   head/chief nurse

infirmière *f* **visiteuse; infirmière visitante**   district nurse; visiting nurse
infirmité *f*   infirmity
inflammation *f*   inflammation
inflammatoire *adj*   inflammatory
influx *m*   influx
- influx nerveux = (nerve) impulse
infrarouge *adj*   infrared
inhalateur *m*   inhaler
- inhalateur buccal = mouth inhaler
- inhalateur de poche = pocket-size inhaler
inhalation *f*   inhalation
inhaler *v*   to inhale; to breathe in
inhibiteur *m*; **inhibiteur, inhibitrice** *adj*   inhibitor; inhibitory *(adj)*
- inhibiteur de la coagulation = inhibitor of coagulation (of blood)
injecté,-e *adj*   injected
injecté (de sang)   bloodshot (eyes)
injecter *v*   to inject
injection *f*   injection
- injection intradermique = intradermal/intradermic injection
- injection intramusculaire = intramuscular injection
- injection intraveineuse = intravenous injection
- injection sous-cutanée = subcutaneous injection
inoculation *f*   1 inoculation; 2 infection
- inoculation accidentelle = infection
inoculer *v*   to inoculate
- inoculer un malade contre ..... = to inoculate a patient against .....
insémination *f* **artificielle avec donneur; IAD**   artificial insemination by donor;
AID
insolation *f*   sunstroke
- attraper une insolation = to get sunstroke
- elle a une insolation = she has got sunstroke
insomniaque *m,f*; **also** *adj*   insomniac
insomnie *f*   insomnia
- j'ai des insomnies = I have insomnia; I can't sleep
instiller *v*   to instil
insuffisance *f*   insufficiency; inadequacy
- insuffisance cardiaque = cardiac insufficiency
- insuffisance hépatique = liver failure; hepatic insufficiency
- insuffisance renale = renal insufficiency
- insuffisance respiratoire = respiratory insufficiency
- insuffisance(s) thyroïdienne(s) = thyroid insufficiency

insuffisant,-e *adj*; **insuffisant** *m*   insufficient; inadequate; insufficient person
- insuffisant cardiaque/rénal = person suffering from cardiac/renal insufficiency
- les insuffisants respiratoires = people with respiratory insufficiency

insufflateur *m*   insufflator
insufflation *f*   insufflation
insuffler *v*   to blow; to insufflate
insuline *f*   insulin
- choc insulinique = insulin shock
- insulinothérapie f = insulin treatment

interféron *m*   interferon
intermission *f*   intermission
intermittence *f*   1 remission; 2 irregularity (eg of heart); 3 intermittence; intermittency
internat *m*   hospital training; period as houseman or intern; entrance examination (for hospital work)
- pendant son internat = during his/her period as an intern

interne *m,f* **(des hôpitaux)**   house doctor; houseman
interné *m*; **internée** *f*   inmate (eg of a mental hospital)
interne *adj*   internal; interior
internement *m*   confinement (eg to a mental hospital)
interner *v*   to intern (eg in a psychiatric hospital)
interrompre *v*   to interrupt; to break off; to terminate
- interrompre une grossesse = to terminate a pregnancy

interruption *f* **(volontaire) de grossesse; IVG**   abortion
intervenir *v*   to intervene; to operate
- le chirurgien a décidé d'intervenir = the surgeon has decided to operate

intervention *f*   intervention; operation
- il vient de subir une petite intervention = he has just had a minor operation
- une intervention chirurgicale = surgical operation

intestin *m*   intestine
- intestins = bowels
- syndrome de l'intestin irritable = irritable bowel syndrome

intestin *m* **grêle**   small intestine; bowel
intestin *m* **, gros**   large intestine
intoxication *f*   poisoning
intoxication *f* **alimentaire**   food poisoning
intoxiqué *m*; **intoxiquée** *f*   drug addict
intoxiquer *v*   to poison
intubation *f*   intubation
intuber *v*   to intubate
invalide *m,f*; **also** *adj*   disabled person; disabled *(adj)*

involutif,-ive *adj* involute
 ▪ processus involutif = involution
involution *f* involution
iridocyclite *f* iridocyclitis
iris *m* iris (eye)
iritis *m* [AM: inflammation de l'iris] iritis [AM: inflammation of the iris]
irradiation *f* irradiation; radiation
irréductible *adj* **(par ex. hernie)** irreducible (eg hernia)
irrégulier *adj* anomalous
irrigateur *m* irrigator (appliance)
irrigation *f* irrigation
irriguer *v* to irrigate
irritant *m*; **irritant,-e** *adj* irritant
irritation *f* **(syn. excitation)** irritation
isolement *m* isolation
 ▪ hôpital d'isolement = isolation hospital

J

jambe *f* leg
 ▪ jambe articulée = articulated leg
 ▪ jambe artificielle = artificial leg
jarret *m* back of the knee
jaunisse *f* (syn. ictère) jaundice
jéjunum *m* [AM: partie de l'intestin grêle] jejunum [AM: part of small intestine]
jeun; à jeun *adv* on an empty stomach
 ▪ à prendre à jeun = to be taken on an empty stomach
jeûne *m* fasting; abstention from food
jeûner *v* to fast
jogging *m* jogging
 ▪ aller faire un jogging = to go jogging
 ▪ faire son jogging quotidien = to go for one's daily jog
joue *f* cheek
jumeaux *mpl*; **jumeau** *m*; **jumelle** *f* twins; twin (male, female)

K

Kaposi, sarcome de Kaposi's sarcoma
kératine *f* keratin
kératite *f* [AM: inflammation de la cornée] keratitis [AM: inflammation of the cornea]
kiné *m,f* physio; physiotherapist
kinésithérapeute *m,f* physiotherapist; physical therapist
kinésithérapie *f* physiotherapy
kleptomanie *f* kleptomania
kyste *m* cyst
kyste *m* **sébacé; (syn: loupe)** sebaceous cyst
kystique *adj* cystic

L

L-dopa *f* [AM: utilisée dans le traitement de la maladie de Parkinson] L-dopa [AM: used in treatment of Parkinson's disease]
laboratoire *m* laboratory
- laboratoire biochimique = biochemical laboratory
- laboratoire de virologie = virology laboratory
- laboratoire pathologique = pathological laboratory
- laboratoire physiologique = physiological laboratory
- laboratoire radiochimique = radiochemical laboratory
lactation *f* lactation
lait m 1 milk; 2 lotion
- lait démaquillant = cleansing lotion
- lait de toilette = cleansing lotion; cleansing milk
- lait de toilette pour bébés = baby lotion
- lait pour le corps = body lotion
lame *f* **de rasoir** razor blade
lancette *f* lancet
langue *f* tongue
- avoir la langue blanche/chargée = to have a coated or furred tongue
- ouvrez la bouche; tirez la langue = open your mouth; put your tongue out
lanoline *f* **(graisse de laine)** lanolin
laparotomie *f* [AM: ouverture de la cavité abdominale] laparotomy [AM: opening the abdominal cavity]
laque *f***; bombe** *f* **de laque** hair spray

laryngectomie *f* [AM: ablation de la totalité ou une partie du larynx] laryngectomy [AM: removal of part or whole of larynx]

laryngite *f* [AM: inflammation du larynx] laryngitis [AM: inflammation of the larynx]

laryngoscope *m* laryngoscope

laryngoscopie *f* [AM: examen visuel du larynx à l'aide d'un laryngoscope] laryngoscopy [AM: visual examination of larynx using a laryngoscope]

larynx *m* larynx

laser *m* laser

lassitude *f* lassitude

lavage *m* washing; washing out
- faire un lavage d'estomac à quelqu'un = to pump someone's stomach out
- lavage d'intestin = intestinal wash
- lavage gastrique = stomach wash

lavage *m* **interne** douche

lavement *m* enema; rectal injection
- lavement baryté = barium enema (for radiological examination)

laver *v* to wash out (eg the intestine)

laxatif *m*; **laxatif,-ive** *adj* laxative

lentigo *m* mole; lentigo

lentilles *fpl* **de contact** contact lenses

lèpre *f* leprosy

lesbianisme *m* lesbianism

lesbienne *f*; **also** *adj* lesbian

léser *v* to damage; to injure

lésion *f* lesion
- lésion pulmonaire = pulmonary lesion
- lésions cérébrales = brain damage
- lésions internes = internal injuries

léthargie *f* lethargy

leucémie *f* leukaemia; leukemia

leucocyte *m* **(syn. globule blanc)** leucocyte [AM: white blood cell]

leucorrhée *f* **(syn. pertes blanches)** leukorrhea; leucorrhea

leucotomie *f* **(syn. lobotomie)** leucotomy

lèvre *f* lip
- commissures des lèvres = corners of the lips/mouth
- les lèvres d'une plaie/incision = the edges of a wound/incision
- lèvre supérieure/inférieure = upper/lower lip

libérer *v* to unblock (eg intestine)

libido *f* libido

licenciement *m* discharge (of patient)

ligament *m* ligament

ligature *f* ligature
ligaturer *v* to ligature; to tie up; to bind (eg arterey)
limaçon *m* **osseux** **(syn. cochlée)** cochlea
lime *f* **à ongles** nailfile
lingettes *fpl* baby wipes
linguette *f* under-tongue tablet
lipide *m* lipid
liposoluble *adj* liposoluble; fat soluble
liposuccion *f* liposuction
liquide *m* **amniotique** amniotic fluid
liquide *m* **synovial** synovial fluid; synovial liquid
listériose *f* listeriosis; listeria
lit *m* bed
  ▪ lit d'eau = water bed
  ▪ lit privé = private bed
lithiase *f* **rénale** nephritic lithiasis
lithiase *f* **urinaire** gravel; urinary calculus
lobe *m* **de l'oreille** ear lobe
lobe *m* **inférieur** lower lobe (lung)
lobe *m* **moyen** middle lobe (lung)
lobe *m* **supérieur** upper lobe (lung)
lobotomie *f* **cérébrale** leucotomy; lobotomy
lobule *m* lobule; ear lobe
local *m* **d'examens** examination room
lombaire *adj* lumbar
  ▪ dans la région lombaire = in the lumbar region
lombalgie *f* lumbago
longévité *f* longevity
lordose *f* lordosis
lotion *f* lotion
  ▪ lotion après-rasage = aftershave
  ▪ lotion après-soleil = after-sun lotion
  ▪ lotion avant-rasage = pre-shave lotion
  ▪ lotion calmante à la calamine = calamine lotion
  ▪ lotion capillaire = hair lotion
  ▪ lotion contre les insectes = insect repellant
  ▪ lotion pré-rasage = pre-shave lotion
loupe *f* **(syn. kyste sébacé)** 1 sebaceous cyst; 2 wen; 3 magnifying glass
luette *f* uvula
lumbago *m* lumbago
lunettes *fpl* glasses

- lunettes bifocales = bifocal glasses
- lunettes de protection = safety goggles
- lunettes de sécurité = safety glasses
- lunettes de soleil = sunglasses
- lunettes noires = dark glasses

lupus *m* **érythémateux aigu disséminé** systemic acute lupus erythematosis
lupus *m* **érythémateux chronique** chronic lupus erythematosis
lupus *m* **(vulgaire)** lupus (vulgaris)
luxation *f* dislocation
luxer *v* to dislocate
lymphangite *f* lymphangitis
lymphatique *adj* lymphatic
- système lymphatique = lymphatic system

lymphe *f* lymph
lymphosarcome *m* lymphosarcoma

M

mâchoire *f* jaw
- mâchoire inférieure/supérieure = lower/upper jaw

mâchonnement *m* bruxism (grinding of teeth); chewing
mâchonner *v* to chew
macule *f* macula (discolouration spot)
magnésium *m* magnesium
maigre *adj* underweight; thin
maigrir *v* to slim
- elle suit un régime pour maigrir = she is on a slimming programme
- suivre un régime amaigrissant = to be on a slimming diet

main *f* hand
- main droite/gauche = right/left hand

maison *f* **de cure** sanatorium
majeur *m* 1 middle finger; 2 person over 18
- être majeur(e) = to be over 18

mal *m* ill; sick; sickness; ache
- ça fait mal = it hurts
- comprimé *m* contre le mal des transports = travel-sickness pill
- j'ai mal au cœur = I feel sick
- j'ai mal aux dents = I have a toothache

- j'ai mal ici = I have a pain here
- mal à la gorge = sore throat
- mal à la tête; mal de tête = headache
- mal à l'estomac; mal d'estomac = stomach ache
- mal aux oreilles; mal d'oreilles = earache
- mal aux reins; mal de reins = backache
- mal de dents = toothache
- mal de dos; maux de dos = back pain
- mal de mer = sea sickness
- mal des transports = travel sickness; motion sickness

malade *m,f* invalid; sick person; patient (eg of doctor)
- grand malade = seriously ill person
- malade imaginaire = hypochondriac
- malade mental = mentally ill person

malade *adj* sick; ill
- être malade = to be ill/sick
- gravement malade = seriously/critically ill

maladie *f* illness; disease; affection
- la maladie = sickness; illness; ill health
- maladie à virus Ebola = Ebola virus disease
- maladie bronzée = Addison's disease
- maladie cardio-vasculaire = cardiovascular disease
- maladie chronique = chronic disease
- maladie contagieuse = contagious illness/disease
- maladie coronarienne = coronary heart disease
- maladie d'Addison = Addison's disease
- maladie de langueur = wasting disease
- maladie de Parkinson = Parkinson's disease
- maladie de peau = skin disease
- maladie du cœur = heart disease
- maladie du légionnaire = legionnaires' disease
- maladie du sommeil = sleeping sickness
- maladie du travail = occupational disease
- maladie héréditaire = hereditary diisease
- maladie infantile; maladie d'enfant = childhood disease or complaint
- maladie infectieuse = infectious disease
- maladie mentale = mental illness
- maladie mortelle = fatal illness/disease
- maladie professionnelle = industrial disease; occupational disease
- maladie rare = rare disease; rare illness.
- maladie sexuellement transmissible = sexually transmitted disease, STD
- maladie tropicale = tropical disease

■ maladie vénérienne = venereal disease, VD

malaise *m*   feeling of sickness or fainting

■ avoir un malaise = to feel faint or dizzy

malaria *f* **(syn. paludisme)**   malaria

malarien,ienne *adj*   malarial

malformation *f*   abnormality

malignité *f*   malignancy

malin, maligne *adj* **(ant. bénin, bénigne)**   malignant

■ tumeur maligne = malignant tumour

mamelon *m*   nipple

mammaire *adj*   mammary

■ abcès mammaire = mammary abcess

■ glandes mammaires = mammary glands

mammographie *f* **(syn. mastographie)** [AM: examen des seins aux rayons X]
   mammography [AM: x-ray examination of breasts]

mammographie f   mammogram

mammoplastie *f* **(syn. mastoplastie; plastie mammaire)**   plastic surgery of the
   breast

manie *f*   mania

manipulation *f*   manipulation

■ manipulation vertébrale = manipulation of the spine

■ obtenu par manipulation génétique = genetically engineered

manucure *f*   manicure

manuel *m* **de premiers soins**   first aid manual

maquillage *m*   1 make-up; 2 making-up

maquiller *v*   to make-up

marasme *m* [AM: carence nutritionnelle menant à l'emaciation progressive]   marasmus
   [AM: nutritional deficiency leading to progressive emaciation]

marcher *v* **en dormant**   to sleepwalk

marqueur *m*   marker; tracer

mascara *m*   mascara

masque *m*   1 mask; 2 face-pack

■ masque à oxygène = oxygen mask

■ masque antirides = antiwrinkle face-pack

■ masque de beauté = face pack

■ masque de beauté à l'argile = mud pack

■ masque de gaze = surgical masque

■ masque de grossesse = chloasma (skin pigmentation)

■ masque hydratant = moisturising face-pack

■ masque respiratoire = respirator mask

massage *m*   massage

- massage cardiaque = cardiac massage

masser *v*   1 to massage; 2 to mass

- se faire masser = to have a massage

masseur *m*; **masseuse** *f*   masseur; masseuse

mastectomie *f* [AM: ablation de la glande mammaire]   mastectomy [AM: removal of mammary gland]

mastite *f*   mastitis

mastoïde *f*; also *adj*   mastoid

- apophyse f mastoïde = mastoid process (protuberance)

mastoïdite *f*   mastoiditis

mastoplastie *f*   plastic surgery of the breast

matelas *m*   mattress

- matelas à eau = water mattress
- matelas pneumatique = air mattress; air bed

matière *f*   matter

- matières fécales = faeces

matrice *f* (syn. **utérus**)   uterus; womb

- descente f de matrice = prolapse of the uterus

maturation *f*   maturation

mauvaise haleine *f* (syn. **halitose**)   halitosis; bad breath

maxillaire *m*   jawbone; maxilla

- maxillaire inférieur/supérieur = lower/upper jawbone

maxillaire *adj*   maxillary

mécanicien-dentiste *m*   dental technician; dental mechanic

mèche *f*   pack; dressing

mèche *f*   tent (surgery); wick; pack

- introduire une meche dans une plaie = to tent a wound

mécher *v*   to pack with gauze

médecin *m*   doctor; physician

- médecin accoucheur = obstetrician
- médecin-conseil = medical adviser
- médecin de famille = general practitioner; family doctor
- médecin de garde = doctor on duty; duty doctor
- médecin d'hôpital = consultant
- médecin du travail = company doctor
- médecin légiste = forensic scientist; forensic surgeon
- médecin généraliste = general practitioner (G.P.); family doctor
- médecin militaire = army medical officer
- médecin scolaire = school doctor

médecine *f*   medicine

- médecine alternative/douce/naturelle = alternative medicine

méningite

- médecine curative = remedial medicine
- médecine d'urgence = emergency treatment
- médecine d'urgence (service) = casualty (department)
- médecine du travail = occupational or industrial medicine
- médecine générale = general medicine
- médecine infantile = paediatrics
- médecine légale = forensic medicine
- médecine naturelle = natural medicine
- médecine par les plantes = herbal medicine
- médecine parallèle = complementary medicine
- médecine préventive = preventive medicine
- médecines douces/parallèles = alternative medicine

medical,-e *adj* medical
médicament *m* medicine; drug; remedy

- c'est sans danger pour les enfants? = is it safe to give to children?
- je prends ce médicament = I am taking this medicine
- médicament allopathique = conventional medicine/remedy
- médicament de confort = over-the-counter remedy
- médicament homéopathique = homeopathic medicine/remedy

médicament *m* **contre la stérilité** fertility drug
méditation *f* meditation
mégalomanie *f* megalomania
meilleur; mieux *adj* better

- il s'est très vite remis de sa maladie = he got better very quickly after his illness
- il va/se porte bien mieux maintenant = he is much better now

mélancolie *f* melancholia
mélanine *m* melanin
mélanisme *m* melanism
mélanome *m* melanoma
membrane *f* membrane

- membranule *f* = little membrane
- membrane séreuse = serous membrane

membre *m* limb

- membres supérieurs/inférieurs = upper/lower limbs

memoire *f* memory
Ménière, vertige de, ou maladie de Ménière's disease
méninges *mpl* meninges
méningite *f* meningitis

- méningocoque = meningococcus (micro-organism)

méningite *f* **cérébro-spinale** spinal meningitis

ménopause *f* menopause
ménopausée *adj* post-menopausal
ménopausique *adj* menopausal
ménorragie *f* menorrhagia
menstruation *f* menstruation; menses
menstruel,-elle *adj* menstrual
menton *m* chin
mentonnière *f* chin bandage
mercure *m* mercury
mère *f* **porteuse** surrogate mother
métabolisme *m* metabolism
métacarpe *m* metacarpus
métatarse *m* metatarsus
  ▪ os du métatarse = metatarsals
méthode *f* method
mettre *v* to apply (eg ointment, dressing); to put on
meurtrir *v* to bruise
  ▪ se meurtrir le bras = to bruise one's arm
  ▪ un œil meurtri/une joue meurtrie/des côtes meurtries/un dos meurtri/un muscle
    meurtri = bruised eye/cheek/ribs/back/muscle
microbe *m* microbe; germ
microbiologie *f* microbiology
microbiologiste *m,f* microbiologist
miction *f* micturition
migraine *f* migraine; sick headache
mince *adj* slim; slender
minceur *f* slimness; slenderness
mincir *v* to lose weight
  ▪ régime pour mincir = slimming diet
minerve *f* collar (surgical)
minoxidil *m* [AM: médicament ayant propriétés vasodilatatrices]   minoxidil [AM: vasodilator
    drug]
moelle *f* marrow; medulla [AM: medulla = latin word for marrow]
  ▪ greffe de moelle osseuse = bone marrow transplant
  ▪ moelle épinière = spinal chord; spinal marrow
  ▪ moelle osseuse = bone marrow
molaire *f* molar (tooth)
mollet *m* calf
mongolien *m*; **mongolienne** *f* person with Down's syndrome
mongolien,-ienne *adj* Down's syndrome; with Down's syndrome
mongolisme *m* Down's syndrome; mongolism

moniteur *m* **cardiaque**　heart rate monitor
monitorage *m*　monitoring
monitoring *m*　monitoring
mononucléose *f* **infectieuse**　glandular fever
monstruosité *f*　deformity
morbide *adj*　morbid
morphine *f*　morphine
morsure *f*　bite
- morsure de serpent = snake bite
- une morsure de chien = a dog bite

mort *f*　1 death; 2 dead person
- mort absolue/mort définitive = clinical death
- mort cérébrale/mort clinique/mort relative = brain death
- mort naturelle = natural death
- mort subite imprévue du nourrisson = sudden infant death

morve *f*　glanders
mouchoirs en papier　tissues; paper handkerchiefs
mousse *f* **à raser**　shaving foam
mousse *f* **coiffante**　hair mousse
mousse *f* **pour cheveux**　hair mousse
mucoviscidose *f*　[AM: maladie fibrose kystique du pancréas]　mucoviscidosis　[AM: fibrocystic disease of the pancreas]
muguet *m*　thrush
multiple *adj*　multiple (eg fractures)
muqueuse *f*　mucous membrane
muqueux,-euse *adj*　mucous
muscle *m*　muscle
- muscle biceps brachial = biceps brachii muscle
- muscle biceps crural = biceps femoris muscle
- muscle grand pectoral = pectoralis major muscle
- muscle pectoral = pectoral muscle
- muscle quadriceps crural = quadripeds femoris muscle
- muscles fessiers = gluteal muscles

musculaire *adj*　muscular
musculature *f*　musculature
mutagène *adj*　mutagen; mutagenic
- agent *m* mutagène = mutagen

mutisme *m*　dumbness; muteness; mutism
mutité *f*　dumbness; mutism
mutité *f*　muteness
myasthénie *f*　myasthenia gravis

mycose *f* 1 mycosis; 2 fungus disease
- mycose du pied = athlete's foot
- mycose vaginale = thrush

mycotoxicose *f* mycotoxicosis
mycotoxine *f* mycotoxin
myélite *f* myelitis
myocarde *m* myocardium
myocardite *f* myocarditis
myodynie *f* rheumatism, muscular
myoglobine *f* myoglobin
myopathie *f* myopathy
myopie *f* myopia
myxœdème *m* myxoedema; myxedema

N

nævus *m* nevus; naevus; birthmark; angioma
nanisme *m* dwarfism; nanism
narcose *f* narcosis
narcotique *m*; **also** *adj* drug; narcotic
narine *f* nostril
nasal *adj* nasal
natation *f* swimming
nausée *f* nausea; sick
- j'ai la nausée = I feel sick/nauseous

nausée *f* (du *matin*); **nausées** *fpl* **matinales** morning sickness
nécrose *f* necrosis
néphrite *f* [AM: inflammation du rein] nephritis; acute Bright's disease [AM: inflammation of the kidney]
néphrose *f* nephrosis
nerf *m* nerve
- nerf moteur = motor nerve
- nerf ophtalmique = ophthalmic nerve
- nerf optique = optic nerve
- nerf phrènique = phrenic nerve
- nerf pneumogastrique = vagus nerve; pneumogastric nerve
- nerf rachidien = spinal nerve
- nerf sciatique = sciatic nerve

- nerf sensitif = sensory nerve
- nerf vague = vagus nerve
- nerfs crâniens = cranial nerves
- nerfs spinaux = spinal nerves

nerveux, nerveuse *adj* nervous
- grossesse nerveuse = false pregnancy; phantom pregnancy
- système nerveux = nervous system

nervosité *f* nervousness; nervous tension

neural,-e *adj* neural

neurasthénie *f* neurasthenia; depression

neurasthénique *m,f* depressed person; neurasthenic

neurasthénique *adj* neurasthenic; depressed

neuroleptique *m*; also *adj* neuroleptic

neurologie *f* [AM: étude et traitement du système nerveux] neurology [AM: study and treatment of the nervous system]

neurologique *adj* neurological

neurologue *m,f* neurologist

neuronal,-e *adj* neuronal

neurone *m* neuron

neurone *m* **moteur** motor neuron

neutraliser *v* to neutralise; to block (pain)

névralgie *f* neuralgia

névralgique *adj* neuralgic
- centre/point névralgique = nerve centre

névrite *f* neuritis

névrome *m* [AM: tumeur] neuroma [AM: tumour]

névrose *f* neurosis
- névrose obsessionnelle/phobique = obsessional/phobic neurosis

névrotique *adj* neurotic

nez *m* nose
- avoir le nez bouché = to have a blocked nose

nicotinisme *m* **(syn. tabagisme)** tobacco addiction; nicotine poisoning

nodule *m* nodule

nombril *m* **(syn. ombilic)** navel; umbilicus

noradrénaline *f* noradrenaline

normal,-e *adj* normal

nourrisson *m* new-born baby; (unweaned) infant

nouveau-né,-e *m,f*; also *adj* new-born baby

noyade *f* drowning
- mort *f* par noyade = death by drowning

noyau *m* nucleus

numération f numeration
- numération globulaire = blood count

nuque f nape (of the neck)

nutritif,-ive adj nourishing; nutritive

nutrition f nutrition

nystagmus m nystagmus

O

obèse adj obese

obésité f obesity

oblitérer v to obstruct (eg an artery)

observation f observation
- être/mettre en observation = to be/put under observation

obstétricien m; obstétricienne f obstetrician

obstétrique adj obstetric
- clinique obstétrique = obstetric clinic

obstétrique f midwifery; obstetrics

obstruction f obstruction; blockage

occipital,-e adj occipital
- région occipital = occipital region/area

occiput m occiput

occlure v to occlude

occlusion f occlusion; blockage
- occlusion intestinale = intestinal blockage

oculiste m,f oculist; ophthalmologist; eye specialist
- je cherche un oculiste = I am looking for an optician

odontologie f dentistry

odorat m sense of smell
- il a l'odorat fin = he has a keen sense of smell

œdème m oedema

Œdipe, complex d' Oedipus complex

œil m; yeux mpl eye; eyes

œil m poché; œil au beurre noir black eye

œillère f eyebath; eyecup

œsophage m oesophagus; esophagus; gullet

œstrogène m oestrogen (female hormone)

oignon m 1 bunion; 2 onion

olfaction *f* olfaction
oligurie *f* oliguria
ombilic *m* **(syn. nombril)** navel; umbilicus
ombre *m* **à paupières** eye shadow
omoplate *f* shoulder blade
onctueux,-euse *adj* smooth; creamy
ondulant,-e *adj* uneven (pulse)
ongle *m* nail; fingernail
- ongle de la main = fingernail
- ongle de l'orteil = toenail
- ongle du pied = toenail
- ongle incarné = ingrowing nail
- ongles cassants = brittle nails
- ongles soignés = well-manicured nails
opération *f* operation
- salle d'opération = operating theatre
opératoire *adj* operating (eg methods)
- dépression opératoire = post-operative depression
- maladie opératoire = post-operative illness
opéré *m*; **opérée** *f* patient (who has had an operation)
opérer *v* to operate
- il faudra l'opérer = will he need an operation?
- il va falloir opérer = you will need an operation
- nous devons opérer = we'll have to operate
- on l'a opéré d'une tumeur = he had an operation for a tumour/ to remove a tumour
- se faire opérer = to have an operation
- se faire opérer des amygdales = to have one's tonsils removed
ophtalmie *f* [AM: inflammation de l'œil] ophthalmia [AM: eye inflammation]
ophtalmologie *f* opthalmology
ophtalmologiste *m*; **ophtalmologue** *m* ophthalmologist; eye specialist
ophtalmoscope *m* ophthalmoscope
ophtalmoscopie *f* ophthalmoscopy
opticien *m* optician
oral,-e *adj* oral
oralement *adv* orally
orbite *f* eye-socket; orbit
orchite *f* orchitis
ordinateur *m* **de diagnostic** diagnostic computer
ordonnance *f* prescription
- délivré uniquement sur ordonnance = available on prescription only

- médicament vendu sans ordonnance = over-the-counter medicine
- puis-je l'obtenir sans ordonnance? = can I get it without a prescription?

ordonner *v*   to prescribe

oreille *f*   ear
  - bouchon d'oreille (pour l'eau) = ear plug (for water)
  - boule Quiès ® (pour bruit) = ear plug (for noise)

oreille *f* **externe**   ear, external; auricle

oreille *f* **interne**   ear, internal

oreillette *f*   auricle (heart)

oreillette *f* **droite**   right auricle
  - atrium ; orifice de l'oreillette = atrium

oreillette *f* **gauche**   left auricle

oreillons, les   the mumps

organe *m*   organ
  - organes digestifs = digestive organs
  - organes génitaux = genitalia; genital organs
  - organes génitaux externes/internes = external/internal genital organs

organisme *m*   1 human body; 2 organism; 3 organisation
  - les defénses naturelles de l'organisme = the body's natural defences

orgelet *m*   sty(e)

orteil *m*   toe

orteil *m*, **gros; gros orteil** *m*   big toe

orthodontie *f*   orthodontics

orthopédie *f*   orthopedics

orthopédique *adj*   orthopaedic; orthopedic
  - chirurgie f orthopédique = orthopaedic surgery

orthopédiste *m,f*; **chirurgien** *m*, **chirurgienne** *f* **orthopédiste**   orthopaedic surgeon

orthophonie *f*   speech therapy

os *m*   bone
  - os du carpe = carpals
  - os du métacarpe = metacarpals
  - os iliaque = hip bone

Osgood-Schlatter, maladie d'   Osgood-Schlatter disease

osseux,-euse *adj*   bone; bony

ossification *f*   ossification

ostéite *f*   osteitis

ostéoarthrite *f*   osteoarthritis

ostéopathe *m,f*   osteopath

ostéopathie *f*   osteopathy

ostéoporose *f*   osteoporosis

ostéosarcome *m* osteosarcoma
ostéosclérose *f* osteosclerosis
ostéomyélite *f* osteomyelitis
otite *f* ear infection; otitis; earache
oto-rhino-laryngologie *f* otorhinolaryngology
oto-rhino-laryngologiste *m,f* ear, nose and throat specialist
otologie *f* [AM: étude des maladies de l'oreille] otology [AM: study of diseases of the ear]
ouate *f* cotton wool
 ▪ ouate chirurgicale = surgical cotton wool; surgical cotton
 ▪ ouate hydrophile = cotton wool; absorbent cotton
ouïe *f* hearing
ovaire *m* ovary
overdose *f* overdose (eg drug)
ovulation *f* ovulation
ovule *m* ovum
ovule *m* 1 pessary; 2 vaginal suppository
 ▪ ovule antifongique = antifungus pessary
ovuler *v* to ovulate
oxygène *m* oxygen
 ▪ bouteille d'oxygène = oxgen cylinder; oxygen bottle
oxygénothérapie *f* oxygen therapy
oxyure *m* pinworm; threadworm; seatworm; oxyurid
oxyurose *f* enterobiasis; oxyuriasis

P

pacemaker *m*; (syn. **stimulateur** *m* **cardiaque**) pacemaker
Paget, maladie *f* **cutanée de** Paget's disease; Paget's carcinoma (of nipple)
Paget, maladie *f* **osseuse de** Paget's disease of bone
palais *m* palate
 ▪ palais fendu = cleft palate
pâleur *f* pallor; paleness
palliatif *m*; **palliatif,-ive** *adj* palliative
palpation *f* palpation
palper *m* palpation
palper *v* to palpate
palpitations *fpl* palpitations
paludéen,-enne; paludique; palustre *adj* paludal; malarial

paludisme *m*   malaria; paludism
panaris *m*   whitlow
pancréas *m*   pancreas
pancreatite *f*   pancreatitis
pancréatique *adj*   pancreatic
pansement *m*   dressing; bandage
- mettre un pansement/un bandage à/sur = to dress (wound etc)
- pansement adhésif = adhesive plaster
- pansement compressif = compressive bandage
- pansement sec/humide = dry/moist dressing

panser *v*   1 to dress (a wound); 2 to put a dressing on; 3 to bandage ; 4 to fill temporarily (tooth)
papier *m* **hygiénique**   toilet paper
papier *m* **toilette**   toilet paper
papilles *fpl* **linguales; papilles** *fpl* **gustatives**   taste buds; lingual papillae
papule *f*   papule
papulo-pustule *f*   papulo-pustule
paracétamol *m* [AM: analgésique et antipyrétique]   paracetamol [AM: analgesic and antipyretic]
paralysé *m*; **paralysée** *f*   paralytic; paralysed man, woman
paralyser *v*   to paralyse; to paralyze
paralysie *f*   palsy; paralysis
- paralysie agitante = shaking palsy
- paralysie faciale = facial paralysis
- paralysie infantile = infantile paralysis; poliomyelitis

paramédical,-e *adj*   paramedical
paranoïa *f*   paranoïa
paraphimosis *m*   paraphimosis
paraplégie *f*   paraplegia
paraplégique *m,f*; **also** *adj*   paraplegic
parasite *m*   parasite
parasitique *adj*   parasitic
parathyroïde *f*   parathyroid; parathyroid gland
paratyphoïde *f*   paratyphoid; paratyphoid fever
parésie *f*   paresis; partial paralysis
parfum m   1 perfume; scent; 2 flavour
parisitaire *adj*   parasitic
Parkinson, maladie de   Parkinson's disease
parodontite *f*   periadontitis
paroi *f*   wall (eg of stomach)
parotidite *f*   parotiditis

paroxysme *m*   paroxysm
pastille *f* **pour la toux**   cough lozenge; cough tablet
pastilles *fpl* **pour la gorge**   throat pastilles
patch *m* **à la nicotine**   nicotine patch
patch-test *m*   patch-test
pâte *f* **dentifrice**   toothpaste
pathogène *adj*   pathogenic
  ▪ agent pathogène = pathogen
pathologie *f*   pathology
pathologique *adj*   pathological
pathologiste *m,f*   pathologist
patient *m*; **patiente** *f*   patient
paume *f*   palm
paupière *f*   eyelid
  ▪ paupière inférieure/supérieure = lower/upper eyelid
pavillon *m* **auriculaire**   auricle (ear)
pavillon *m* **de l'oreille**   auricle; external ear
peau *f*   skin
  ▪ peau grasse/sèche = greasy/dry skin
  ▪ peau morte = scurf; dead skin
  ▪ peau relâchée = slack/loose skin
pectoral,-e *adj*   pectoral; chest
  ▪ sirop pectoral = cough syrup
  ▪ muscles pectoraux = pectoral muscles
pédiatre *m,f*   paediatrician; pediatrician
pédiatrie *f*   paediatrics; pediatrics
pédiculose *f*   pediculosis; infestation with lice
pédicure *m,f*   chiropodist; podiatrist (US)
pédologie *f*   paedology; pedology
peeling *m*   skin peeling treatment
peigne *m*   comb
  ▪ peigne à poux = fine-tooth comb (for headlice)
pelade *f*   [AM: chute des cheveux]   alopecia areata   [AM: hair loss]
pellagre *f*   pellagra
pellicules *fpl*   dandruff
  ▪ lotion contre les pellicules = dandruff lotion
pelvis *m* **(syn. bassin)**   pelvis
pénicilline *f*   penicillin
  ▪ je suis allergique à la pénicilline = I am allergic to penicillin
pénis *m* **(syn. verge)**   penis
pepsine *f*   pepsin

percer *v* to lance; to burst (eg abcess, boil)
percussion *f* percussion; percussion massage
percutané,-e *adj* percutaneous
percuter *v* to percuss
perforateur *m* perforator
perforation *f* perforation
perforer *v* to perforate
perfusion *f* drip; IV (US); perfusion
  ▪ mettre quelqu'un sous perfusion = to put someone on a drip or an IV (US)
périarthrite *f* periarthritis
péricarde *m* pericardium
péricardite **f** pericarditis
périnée *m* perineum
période *f* d'incubation incubation period
périodique *adj* recurring (eg fever); periodic
péristaltisme *m* peristalsis
péritoine *m* peritonium
péritonite *f* peritonitis
perlèche *f* [AM: inflammation des commissures des lèvres] **perleche** [AM: inflammation of the corners of the lips]
pernicieux,-ieuse *adj* pernicious
péroné *m* fibula (leg bone)
peroxyde *m* peroxide
  ▪ eau oxygénée = hydrogen peroxide
perspiration *f* perspiration
perte *f* loss; losing (eg blood)
  ▪ perte de connaissance = loss of consciousness, fainting
  ▪ perte de mémoire = loss of memory, memory loss
  ▪ pertes blanches = vaginal discharge, leucorrhœa
  ▪ pertes de sang = heavy bleeding
pessaire *m* pessary
peste *f* plague
petit mal *m* **épileptique** petit mal; minor epilepsy
pétrir *v* to knead
pétrissage petrissage; kneading massage
phalange *f* phalanx (*pl* phalanges) (finger bone)
pharmacie *f* chemist's; pharmacy
  ▪ pharmacie de garde = night pharmacy; pharmacy in service; pharmacy that's open
pharmacien *m*; **pharmacienne** *f* pharmacist
pharmacologie *f* pharmacology

pharyngite *f* pharyngitis
pharynx *m* pharynx
phase *f* phase; stage
phlébite *f* phlebitis
phobie *f* phobia
phosphore *m* phosphorus
photophobie *f* [AM: crainte de la lumière] photophobia [AM: aversion to light]
photosensibilisation *f* photosensitization
physiologie *f* physiology
physiothérapeute *m,f* physiotherapist
physiothérapie *f* physiotherapy
phytothérapeute *m,f* herbalist
phytothérapie *f* herbal medicine
pian *m* yaws; pian
pied *m* foot
  ▪ mycose du pied = athlete's foot
  ▪ pied bot = club-foot; talipes
  ▪ pied creux = hollow foot; pes cavus
  ▪ pied plat = flat foot; pes valgus
pierre *f* stone
pierreux,-euse *adj* calculous
pigment *m* pigment
pigmentation *f* pigmentation
pilule *f* pill
  ▪ minipilule *f* = minipill
pilule *f* **anticonceptionnelle; pilule contraceptive** contraceptive pill
  ▪ j'ai arrêté la pilule = I have come off the pill
  ▪ je prends la pilule = I am on the pill
pilule *f* **du lendemain** morning-after pill
pince *f* **à cheveux** hairclip; hair grip
pince *f* **à échardes** tweezers
pince *f* **à épiler** tweezers (eyebrow)
pince *f* **à ongles** nail clippers
pincement *m* pinch; pinching massage
pincer *v* to pinch
pinçon *m* pinch mark; blood blister
piquer *v* to give an injection ; to give a jab; to sting (insect)
  ▪ il s'est fait piquer par une méduse = he was stung by a jellyfish
  ▪ je me suis fait piquer par une guêpe = I have been stung by a wasp
  ▪ se faire piquer contre la variole = to have a smallpox injection
piqûre *f* 1 sting; bite (of insect); 2 injection

- piqûre d'abeille/de guêpe = bee/wasp sting
- piqûre de méduse = jellyfish sting
- piqûre de rappel; rappel *m* = booster shot; booster dose
- piqûre d'insecte = insect bite
- se faire faire une piqûre = to have an injection

pituitaire *f*; **also** *adj* pituitary

placebo *m* placebo

placenta *m* placenta; afterbirth

plaie *f* sore; wound

planification *f* **familiale; planning** *m* **familial** family planning

plante *f* **(du pied)** sole (of the foot)

plaque *f* **dentaire** dental plaque

plaquettes *fpl* **sanguines** blood platelets

plasma *m* **sanguin** blood plasma

plat,-e *adj* flat
- avoir les pieds plats = to have flat feet

plâtre *m* plaster
- mettre dans le plâtre = to put/set in plaster

pleurésie *f* pleurisy

pleurétique *adj* pleuritic

plèvre *f* pleura

plexus *m* plexus

plexus *m* **cardiaque** cardiac plexus

plombage *m* filling (tooth)
- j'ai perdu un plombage = I have lost a filling
- le plombage est parti = the filling has come out
- un plombage a sauté = a filling has fallen out

pneumoconiose *f* pneumoconiosis

pneumocoque *m* pneumococcus

pneumonie *f* **(syn. fluxion de poitrine)** pneumonia
- pneumonie virale = viral pneumonia

pneumonie *f* **des légionnaires** legionnaires' disease

podologie *f* chiropody; podiatry (US)

poids *m* weight

poignet *m* wrist

poil *m* hair (body)

poing *m* fist

point *m* point; place; spot
- avoir le point de côté = to have the stitch
- avoir un point dans le dos = to have a twinge (of pain) in one's back
- avoir un point de côté = to have a stitch in one's side

posologie

- faire des points de suture à = to put stitches in; to stitch up
- point aveugle = blind spot
- point de côté = stitch [AM: pain in the side]
- point de suture = stitch
- point névralgique = nerve centre
- point noir (visage) = blackhead (face) (see comédon m)
- vous avez un point de congestion là = you have a spot of congestion there

pointe *f* point; tip

poison *m* poison

poitrine *f* chest; breasts

- je ressens une douleur dans la poitrine = I have a pain in my chest

poliomyélite *f* poliomyelitis

pollution *f* pollution

- pollutions nocturnes = wet dreams; nocturnal emissions

polyarthrite *f* polyarthritis

polyarthrite *f* **chronique évolutive; PCE** rheumatoid arthritis

polyarthrite *f* **rhumatoïde** rheumatoid arthritis

polymyosite *f* polymyositis

polynévrite *f* polyneuritis

polype *m* polyp; polypus

polyvalent,-e *adj* polyvalent (eg serum, vaccine)

pommade *f* ointment

- pommade antibiotique = antibiotic ointment
- pommade anti-infection = disinfecting ointment; germicidal ointment
- pommade contre les brûlures = ointment for burns
- pommade pour les lèvres = lip salve
- pommade rosat = lip-salve

pomme *f* **d'Adam** Adam's apple

pommette *f* cheekbone

pompe *f* **stomacale** stomach pump

ponction *f* puncture

- ponction lombaire = lumbar puncture

pontage *m* bypass; bypass operation

- pontage cardiaque = (heart) bypass operation
- pontage coronarien = coronary bypass

porphyrie *f* porphyria

porteur *m,f* carrier

- porteur de germes = germ carrier

pose *f* **d'une prothèse de la hanche** hip replacement operation

posologie *f* dosage

post-cure *f* aftercare (eg convalescent care)
post-opératoire *adj* post-operative
posture *f* posture
pot *m* **(d'enfant)** child's chamber pot; potty
potassium *m* potassium
Pott, mal *m* **de** Pott's disease
pou *m*; **poux** *mpl* louse; lice (pl); pediculus
  ▪ avoir des poux = to have lice
pouce *m* thumb
poudre *f* powder
  ▪ poudre dentifrice = tooth powder
  ▪ poudre de riz = face powder
poudrier *m* powder compact
pouls *m* pulse
  ▪ le rhythme du pouls est d'environ 70 battements à la minute = the pulse rate is about 70 beats a minute
  ▪ prendre le pouls de quelqu'un = to take someone's pulse
poumon *m* lung
  ▪ abcés du poumon = an abcess of the lung
  ▪ poumon gauche/droit = left/right lung
Pouteau-Colles, fracture de Colles' fracture
praticien *m*; **praticienne** *f* practitioner
pratiquer *v* to practise; to carry out
prééclampsie *f* pre-eclampsia
prélèvement *m* sample; sampling
  ▪ faire un prélèvement de sang = to take a blood sample
  ▪ je voudrais un prélèvement de votre sang/de vos selles/de votre urine = I would like a specimen of your blood/ stools/ urine
prélever *v* to take (eg sample)
  ▪ prélever sur = to remove from
  ▪ prélever un échantillon de = to take a sample of (eg blood)
  ▪ prélever un organe = to remove an organ
premiers soins *mpl* first aid
prendre *v* to take; to catch (eg a cold)
  ▪ à prendre avant les repas = to be taken before meals
  ▪ à prendre matin, midi et soir = to be taken three times a day
  ▪ à prendre trois fois par jour = to be taken three times a day
  ▪ prendre un rhume = to catch a cold
préopératoire *adj* preoperative
prépuce *m* prepuce
presbytie *f* presbyopia; longsightedness

prescription *f* prescription; directions
- se conformer aux prescriptions du medecin = to be taken in accordance with doctors' instructions

prescrire *v* to prescribe
- ne pas dépasser la dose prescrite = do not exceed the prescribed dose

présentation *f* presentation
- présentation par la tête/le siège = head/breech presentation (of baby)

présenter *v* to present

préservatif *m* condom

pression *f* pressure
- pression artérielle = blood pressure
- pression (artérielle) diastolique/systolique = diastolic/systolic blood pressure
- pression intraoculaire = intraocular pressure
- pressions = pressure massage

prévention *f* prevention

priapisme *m* priapism

primaire *adj* primary

pris, prise *adj* taken; affected
- j'ai la gorge prise = my throat is hoarse
- j'ai le nez pris = my nose is stuffed up

prise *f* **de sang** blood sample; taking a blood sample

produit m
- produit antimoustique = mosquito repellent
- produit contre l'acné = antiacne cream/lotion
- produit pharmaceutique = pharmaceutical product

progestérone *f* progesterone

prolapsus *m* prolapse

prompts secours *mpl* first aid

pronostic *m* prognosis

prophylaxie *f* prophylaxis

prostaglandine *f* prostaglandin

prostate *f* prostate
- cancer de la prostate = prostate cancer

prostatectomie *f* [AM: ablation partielle ou totale de la prostate] prostatectomy
[AM: partial or total removal of the prostate]

prostatite *f* prostatitis

prostration *f* prostration

protection *f* **contre les maladies** health care

protection f maternelle et infantile heath care for mothers and young children

protège-slip *m* panty liner

protège-tympan *m* ear plugs
proteine *f* protein
prothèse *f* prosthesis
- prothèse acoustique = hearing aid
- prothèse auditive = hearing aid
- prothèse de la hanche = hip replacement
- prothèse dentaire = denture
- prothèse valvulaire = artificial heart valve

prurit *m* itching; pruritus
prématuré *m*; **prématuré,-ée** *adj* premature (baby)
psittacose *f* [AM: maladie transmise par les oiseaux (perruche, perroquet)] psittacosis [AM: infection transmitted by birds (budgerigar, parrot]
psoas *m*; **muscle psoas-iliaque** iliopsoas muscle
psoriasis *m* [AM: maladie cutanée] psoriasis [AM: skin disease]
psychanalyse *f* psychoanalysis
psychanalyste *m,f* psychoanalyst
psychiatre *m,f* psychiatrist
psychiatrie *f* psychiatry
psychiatrique *adj* psychiatric
psychologie *f* psychology
psychologique *adj* psychological
psychologue *m,f* psychologist
psychopathe *m,f*; **also** *adj* psychopath
psychopathie *f* psychopathy
psychose *f* psychosis
psychothérapie *f* psychotherapy
puberté *f* puberty
pubien,-ienne *adj* pubic
pubis *m* pubis
- poils *mpl* du pubis = pubic hair

puéricultrice *f* paediatric nurse, paediatric
puerpéral,-e *adj* puerperal
pulmonaire *adj* pulmonary
pulpe dentaire *f* dental pulp
pulsation *f* pulsation; beat (eg heart)
- le rythme cardiaque normal varie de 60-100 pulsations/minute = the normal heartbeat varies between 60-100 beats/minute

pulvérisation *f* pulverization; spray(ing)
- le médecin a ordonné des pulvérisations (nasales) = the doctor prescribed a nasal spray

pupille *f* pupil (eye)

purgatif *m*; **purgatif,-ive** *adj*   purgative
purgation *f*   purgation; purgative
purge *f* (colloq)   purgative
purge *f*   purge; purgative
purger *v*   to purge
purpura *m*   purpura
pus *m*   pus
pustule *f*   pustule
pustulose *f*   pustulosis
pylore *m*   pylorus
pyorrhée *f* **alvéolaire**   pyorrhea
pyrogène *adj*   pyrogenic

Q

quarantenaire *adj*   quarantine
quinine *f*   quinine
Quinke, œdème de   angioneurotic oedema [AM: severe allergic hives]
quinte *f* **de toux**   coughing fit
quotient *m* **intellectuel; quotient d'intelligence**   intelligence quotient; IQ

R

rachis *m*   vertebral column
rachitique *adj*   rachitic
rachitisme *m*   rickets; rachitis
 ▪ être rachitique = to have rickets; to suffer from rickets
racine *f*   root
 ▪ racine dentaire/d'une dent = root (of a tooth)
racler *v*   to scrape
radiation *f* **ionisante**   ionizing radiation
radical *m* **libre**   free radical
radioactif,-ive *adj*   radioactive
radioactivité *f*   radioactivity
radiographe *m*   radiologist

radiographie *f*; **radio** *f* radiography; x-ray photography; radiograph
- il faut vous faire une radio = you will need to have an X-ray taken
- passer une radio des poumons = to have a chest/lung x-ray
- passer une radiographie = to have an x-ray taken

radiographier *v* to x-ray
- se faire radiographier = to have an x-ray taken

radiologie *f* radiology

radiologue *m,f* radiologist

radiologiste *m,f* radiologist

radioscopie *f* fluoroscopy

radiothérapeute *m,f* radiotherapist

radiothérapie *f* radiotherapy (eg x-ray treatment)

radius *m* [AM: os de l'avant-bras] radius [AM: bone of forearm]

rage, la rabies; hydrophobia
- vaccination antirabique = antirabies vaccination

rage *f* **de dents** toothache

raie *f* **des fesses** anal cleft

râle *m* rale (breathing noises); groan

ramoir *v* to soften

ramollissement *m* softening

ramollissement *m* **cérébral (syn. infarctus cérébral)** stroke; cerebrovascular accident

rappel *m* booster (eg vaccination); recall; reminder

raser *v* to shave

rash *m* rash

rasoir *m* razor
- rasoir à piles = battery shaver
- rasoir de sûreté = safety razor
- rasoir électrique = electric shaver
- rasoir jetable = disposable razor
- rasoir mécanique = razor; safety razor

rate *f* spleen

raviver *v* to reopen (eg wound); to revive (eg grief)

Raynaud, maladie de [AM: troubles vasomoteurs des extrémités] Raynaud's disease [AM: vascular spasm of extremities]

rayonnant,-e *adj* spreading (eg pain)

rayonnement m infrarouge infrared radiation

rayonnement *m* **ultraviolet** ultraviolet radiation

rayons *mpl* **gamma** gamma rays

rayons *mpl* **ultraviolets** ultraviolet radiation

réaction *f* reaction

- cuti-réaction f = skin test; Heaf test
- virage d'une cuti-réaction = positive reaction of a skin test

réadaptation *f* **physique**   physical rehabilitation
réadapter *v*   to rehabilitate; to readjust
réanimateur *m*   1 resuscitator; 2 respirator
réanimation *f*   resuscitation
réanimation *f*   1 intensive care; 2 resuscitation
- être en réanimation = to be in intensive care
- service de la réanimation = intensive care unit

réanimer *v*; **ranimer** *v*   to resuscitate
réceptivité *f*   sensitivity; liability; receptivity
- réceptivité à = sensitivity to

récessif,-ve *adj*   recessive
receveur *m*   recipient
- receveur universel = universal recipient

receveuse *f*   recipient
recherche *f* **du groupe sanguin**   blood grouping
rechute *f*   relapse
- faire/avoir une rechute = to have a relapse

rechuter *v*   to relapse; to have a relapse
récidivant,-e *adj*   recurring
récidive *f*   recurrence
récidiver *v*   to recur
récidivité *f*   recurring nature
recoudre *v*   to stitch up; to stitch up again; to put stitches back in (eg wound)
rectal,-e *adj*   rectal
rectite *f*   rectitis
rectoscope *m*   rectoscope
rectoscopie *f*   rectoscopy
rectum *m*   rectum; back passage
récupération *f*   recovery: recuperation
récupérer *v*   to recover; to recuperate
récurrent,-e *adj*   recurrent
réductible *adj*   reductible
réduction *f*   reduction; setting (eg of a fracture)
réduire *v*   to set; to reduce (eg fracture)
rééducation *f*   rehabilitation; physiotherapy
- faire de la rééducation = to undergo/have physiotherapy
- rééducation de la parole = speech therapy

rééduquer *v*   to rehabilitate; to re-educate
réflexologie *f*   reflexology

refroidissement *m*   chill
- prendre un refroidissement = to catch a chill

régime *m*   diet; system; regime
- régime amaigrissant = slimming diet
- régime de la Sécurité sociale = Social Security system
- régime des hôpitaux = hospital system/regulations
- régime maladie = health insurance scheme
- suivre un régime = to be on a diet

règles *fpl*   period; menstruation
- j'ai des règles douloureuses = I have period pains
- je n'ai pas eu mes règles depuis trois mois = I haven't had my period for three months

regonfler *v*   to swell up again

régression *f*   regression

régurgitation *f*   regurgitation

rein *m*   kidney
- avoir mal aux reins = to have backache
- rein droit/gauche = right/left kidney

rein *m* **artificiel (syn. hémodialyseur** *m*)   dialysis machine

rejet *m*   rejection (eg of graft); vomiting

relaxant *m*; **relaxant,-ante** *adj*   relaxant; relaxing

relaxation *f*   relaxation

remboursement *m*   refund; reimbursement

remède *m*   remedy, cure; medicine; ointment
- remède hémorroïdaire = ointment for haemorrhoids

rémission *f*   remission (eg of illness); subsidence; lowering (eg of fever); abatement (eg of pain)

remontant *m*   tonic; antidepressant

remplaçant *m*; **remplaçante** *f*   locum; replacement

rénal,-e *adj*   renal
- défaillance rénale; insuffisance rénale = renal failure
- insuffisance rénale aiguë = acute renal failure

reposer (se) *v*   to rest

résille *f*   hair net

résorber *v*   to resorb

résoudre *v*   to resolve (eg tumour)

respirateur *m*   respirator
- respirateur artificiel = ventilator

respiration *f*   breathing; respiration
- respiration artificielle = artificial respiration
- respiration assistée = assisted ventilation

respiratoire *adj* respiratory
- appareil respiratoire = respiratory tract
- arrêt m respiratoire = respiratory failure
- système respiratoire = respiratory system; respiratory tract

respirer *v* to breathe
- j'ai de la peine à respirer = I have difficulties in breathing
- respirer avec difficulté = to have difficulty breathing
- respirez! = breathe in
- respirez bien fort = take a deep breath

rester *v* to stay; to remain
- rester au lit = to stay in bed

rétablir de (se) *v* to recuperate from

rétention *f* retention (eg of urine)

rétine *f* retina (eye)

rétinite *f* retinitis

rétrécissement *m* contraction (eg of pupil); shrinking; stricture (eg of heart); stenosis
- rétrécissement de la valve aortique = narrowing of the aortic valve

rétrovirus *m* retrovirus

rêve *m* dream

révulsion *f* revulsion

rhésus *m* rhesus
- facteur Rhésus = Rhesus or Rh factor
- rhésus positif/négatif = rhesus (Rh) positive/negative

rhinite *f* **(syn. coryza)** [AM: inflammation des fosses nasales] rhinitis [AM: inflammation of the nose]

rhinopharyngite *f* rhinopharyngitis

rhumatismal *adj* rheumatic

rhumatisme *m* rheumatism
- rhumatisme articulaire = rheumatism in the joints; articular rheumatism
- rhumatisme articulaire aigu = acute articular rheumatism
- rhumatisme chronique polyarticulaire = rheumatoid arthritis

rhumatoïde *adj* rheumatoid

rhumatologie *f* rheumatology

rhumatologiste *m,f*; **rhumatologue** *m,f* rheumatologist

rhume *m*; **rhume simple**; **rhume de cerveau** cold

rhume *m* **(chronique)** catarrh

rhume *m* **des foins** hay fever

riboflavine *f* riboflavin

rickettsiose *f* rickettsiosis

ride *f* wrinkle

rigidité *f* **cadavérique** rigor mortis
ronflement *m*; **ronflements** *mpl* snoring
ronfler *v* to snore
rosacée *f* rosacea
roséole *f* roseola (eruption)
rotateur *m*; **also** *adj* muscle, rotator (muscle)
rotule *f* patella; kneecap
rouge *m* **à lèvres** lipstick
rougeole *f* measles
rougeur *f* rash; redness; red blotch; red patch
ruban *m* **de tissu adhésif** adhesive tape
rubéole *f* rubella; German measles
rupture *f* rupture
  ▪ rupture tendineuse = rupture of a tendon; tearing of a tendon
rythme *m* **cardiaque** heart rate

S

saccharine *f* saccharin
sacrum *m* sacrum
sage-femme *f* midwife
saignée *f* bleeding; blood letting
saignement *f* bleeding
  ▪ saignement de nez = nosebleed
saigner *v* bleed (to)
salive *f* saliva
salle *f* **d'examens** examination room
salle *f* **d'hôpital** ward
salle *f* **d'opérations** operating theatre; operating room
salmonella *f*; **salmonelle** *f* [AM: bactéries] salmonella [AM: bacteria]
salmonellose *f* [AM: infection causée par les salmonelles] salmonellosis [AM: infection due to salmonella]
salpingite *f* [AM: inflammation de 1 la trompe de Fallope; 2 la trompe d'Eustache] salpingitis [AM: inflammation of (usually) 1 Fallopian tube; (sometimes) 2 Eustachian tube]
sanatorium *m* sanatorium
sang *m* blood
sang *m* **contaminé** contaminated blood
sanitaire *adj* health; sanitary

santé *f* health
- santé mentale = mental health
- santé publique = public health

saphène *f* (veine); **also** *adj* saphenous vein; superficial leg vein

sarcoïdose *f* sarcoidosis

sarcome *m* [AM: tumeur maligne] sarcoma [AM: malignant tumour]

saturnisme *m* lead poisoning; plumbism; saturnism

sauna *m* sauna

sauvetage *m* rescue
- cours de sauvetage = life-saving training

savon *m* soap
- savon à barbe = shaving soap
- savon de Marseille = household soap
- savon dermatologique = dermatological soap
- savon de toilette = toilet soap
- savon doux = mild soap
- savon liquide = liquid soap
- savon mou = soft soap
- savon parfumé = scented soap
- savon pour bébés = baby's soap

scalpel *m* scalpel

scanner *m*; **scanneur** *m* 1 scanner; 2 scan
- passer un scanneur = to have a scan

scanographe *m* scanner

scanographie *f* 1 scanning; 2 scan
- passer une scanographie = to have a scan

scapulaire *m*; **also** *adj* shoulder blade; scapula; scapular *(adj)*

scarificateur *m* scarificator

scarifier *v* to scarify

scarlatine *f* scarlet fever; scarlatina

Scheuermann, maladie de [AM: affection dégénérative de la colonne vertébral]
  Scheuermann's disease [AM: degenerative affection of vertebral column]

schizophrène *adj* schizophrenic

schizophrénie *f* schizophrenia

sciatique *f*; **also** *adj* sciatica; sciatic *(adj)*

scintigraphie *f* scintigraphy

sclérodermie *f* scleroderma

sclérose *f* sclerosis
- sclérose artérielle = hardening of the arteries; arteriosclerosis
- sclérose en plaques = multiple sclerosis; disseminated sclerosis
- sclérose multiple = multiple sclerosis

scléroser (se) *v* to become sclerotic

sclérotique *f* **(syn. sclère** *f***)** [AM: membrane qui enveloppe l'œil] sclera; sclerotic [AM: outer membrane of eye]

scorbut *m* scurvy; scorbutus

scotch-test *m* scotch test

scrofule *f* scrofula

scrotal,-e *adj* scrotal

scrotum m scrotum

séborrhée *f* seborrhoea

sébum *m* sebum

sèche-cheveux *m* hairdryer

sécrétion *f* secretion

sédatif *m*; **sédatif,-ive** *adj* sedative

sédation *f* sedation

sédiment *m* sediment

sein *m* breast
  - abcès du sein = abcess of the breast
  - cancer du sein = breast cancer

sel *m* **de Glauber** Glauber's salt (sodium sulfate)

selles *fpl* stools; motions
  - êtes-vous allé à la selle aujourd'hui? = have you had or passed a motion today?

sels *mpl* **de bain** bath salts

semence *f* semen; sperm

sénile *adj* senile

sénilité *f* senility

sens *m* sense

sensation *f* sensation

sensibilisation *f* sensitization; sensitizing

sensibilisé,-e *adj* sensitized

sensibilité *f* sensitivity

sensitif,-ive *adj* sensitive

sentir *v* 1 to feel; 2 to smell (eg perfume)
  - je ne me sens pas bien = I don't feel well

septicémie *f* septicaemia; septicemia; blood poisoning

septicité *f*; **état** *m* **septique** sepsis

sérénité *f* serenity

séreux,-euse *adj* serous

sérieux,-ieuse *adj* serious

seringue *f* syringe

seringue *f* **pour injections** hypodermic syringe

sérum *m* serum

siege

- sérum antidiphtérique = antidiphtheria serum
- sérum antitétanique = antitetanus serum
- sérum antivenimeux = snakebite serum
- sérum physiologique = physiological solution
- sérum sanguin = blood serum

service *m* ward (in hospital); department
- quel service? = which ward?
- service ambulancier = ambulance service
- service d'accouchement = maternity department; obstetric department
- service d'obstétrique = obstetric department; maternity department
- service d'oto-rhino-laryngologie = ear,nose, and throat department
- service de cancer = cancer ward
- service de gastro-entérologie = gastro-enterology department
- service de maternité = maternity ward
- service de maternité; département de maternité = maternity department; obstetric department
- service de pédiatrie = pediatrics ward
- service de radiologie = x-ray department
- service de secours aux victimes de la circulation = traffic accident service
- service gériatrique = geriatric department
- service radiologique = x-ray department
- services médicaux = health care service

serviette *f* **hygiénique; serviette périodique** sanitary towel

séton *m* **(à méche)** [AM: mèche en coton servant de drain une plaie] **seton** [AM: cotton fibre drainage plug in a wound]

sevrage *m* 1 weaning; 2 withdrawal (eg giving up alcohol, drugs etc)
- symptômes de sevrage = withdrawal symptoms

sexe *m* sex

sexologie *f* sexology

sexologue *m,f* sex therapist

sexualité *f* sexuality

sexué,-ée *adj* sexual

sexuel,-elle *adj* sexual

shampooing *m* shampoo
- gel shampooing = shampoo gel

shampooing *m* **pour bébés** baby shampoo

shunt *m* shunt

sibilant,-e *adj* sibilant (whistling)

SIDA; sida; syndrome immunodéficitaire acquis AIDS; aids; acquired immune deficiency syndrome

siege *m* **complet** complete breech presentation; full breech presentation

92

siege *m* **décomplété** frank breech presentation
sifflement *m* whistling; hissing
- sifflement d'oreilles = ringing in the ears; tinnitus
sigmoïde *m*; **also** *adj* sigmoid colon
signe *m* **clinique** clinical sign
silicone *f* silicone
silicose *f* silicosis
sinus *m* sinus
sinusite *f* sinusitis
siphon *m* siphon
sirop *m* **antitussif** cough mixture; cough syrup
sirop *m* **pour la toux** cough syrup; cough mixture
soif *f* thirst
soigner *v* to treat (eg an illness, a person)
soins *mpl* treatment; care; after-treatment
- je voudrai des soins du visage = I would like a facial
- soins corporels/du corp = body care
- soins du cheveux = hair care
- soins du pédicure; soins du pied = chiropody
- soins du visage = facial
- soins du visage = skin care
- soins intensifs = intensive care
- soins médicaux = medical care; health care.
- soins nettoyants = cleansing treatments
solaire *adj* sun
- crème *f* solaire = suntan cream
- huile *f* solaire = suntan oil
- lotion *f* solaire = suntan lotion
solution *f* solution
- solution de rinçage pour les lentilles de contact = rinsing solution for contact lenses
- solution de stérilisation = sterilizing solution
sommeil *m* sleep
somnambule *m,f* sleepwalker
- elle est somnambule = she sleepwalks
somnambulisme *m* sleepwalking
somnifère *adj* soporific
somnifère *m* sleeping pill
somnolence *f* drowsiness; somnolence
sondage *m* catheterization; probing; probe
sonde *f* 1 catheter; 2 probe

- mettre une sonde à quelqu'un = to put a catheter in someone
- sonde à canal central = catheter
- sonde creuse = catheter
- sonde d'alimentation = feeding tube
- sonde gastrique = stomach tube
- sonde urétrale = urethral catheter

sonder *v* to catheterize; to probe
soporifique *adj* soporific
sortie *f* 1 exit; 2 discharge (of patient)
souffle *m* **cardiaque; souffle** *m* **au cœur** cardiac murmur; heart murmur
souffrant,-e *adj* unwell
- être souffrant = to be unwell

souffrir *v* to suffer
soulager *v* to ease; to relieve
sourcil *m* eyebrow
sourd,-e *adj* deaf
sous-alimentation *f* malnutrition
sparadrap *m* adhesive tape (medical); sticking plaster
- sparadrap microporeux = microporous adhesive tape

spasme *m* spasm
- spasme clonique = clonic spasm
- spasme en flexion = epileptic spasm (baby)
- spasme tonique = tonic spasm

spatule *f* spatula
spécialiste *m,f* specialist
spéculum *m* speculum
sperme *m* **(syn. semence)** semen
spermicide *m*; **also** *adj* spermicide
spermogramme *m* semen analysis
sphincter *m* sphincter
sphincter *m* **anal** anal sphincter
sphygmomanomètre *m* **(syn. tensiomètre)** [AM: appareil servant à mesurer la pression artérielle] sphygmomanometer [AM: instrument for measuring blood pressure]
spina-bifida *m* spina bifida
spondylarthrite *f* **ankylosante** ankylosing spondylitis
spondylite *f* [AM: inflammation d'une vertèbre] spondylitis [AM: inflammation of a vertebra]
spondylopathie *f* [AM: toute affection de la colonne vertébrale] spondylopathy [AM: all disease of the spinal column]
spore *f* spore (eg fungus, bacterium)
spray *m* spray
sprue *f* sprue

squame *f* scale; squama
squameux,-euse *adj* squamous; squamose
squelette *m* skeleton
staphylococcie *f* staphylococcia
staphylocoque *m* staphylococcus (bacterium)
▪ staphylocoque doré = staphylococcus aureus
station *f* **thermale** spa
sténose *f* stenosis
steppage *m* steppage gait
stérile *adj* sterile
stérilet *m* coil; IUD; intra-uterine device
stérilisateur *m* sterilizer
stérilisation *f* sterilization
stériliser *v* to sterilize
stérilité *f* sterility
sternum *m* sternum; breast bone
stéroïde *m*; **also** *adj* steroid
▪ stéroïde hormonal = steroidal hormone
stéthoscope *m* stethoscope
stick *m* stick (cosmet)
▪ stick à raser =shaving stick
stigmate *m* stigma; mark; scar
stimulateur *m* **cardiaque; stimulateur artificiel (syn. pacemaker)** pacemaker
stomacal,-e *adj* stomach
stomatite *f* stomatitis
stomatologie *f* [AM: étude des maladies de la bouche et des dents] stomatology [AM: study of diseases of the mouth and teeth]
stomatologiste *m,f*; **stomatologue** *m,f* stomatologist
stomie *f* stomy
strabisme *m* [AM: défaut de la vision] strabismus [AM: eyesight defect]
streptococcie *f* [AM: infection due aux streptocoques] streptococcia [AM: infection by streptococci bacteria]
streptocoque *m* streptococcus (bacterium)
streptomycine *f* streptomycin
stress *m, inv* stress
stressant,-e *adj* stressful
stresser *v* to put under stress
▪ être stressé = to be stressed; to be on edge
stupéfiant *m*; **stupéfiant,-e** *adj* drug; narcotic; stupefying (adj)
stupéfier *v* to stupefy
stupeur *f* stupor

stylet *m* stylet; stilette (small probe)
succion *f* suction; sucking
sucette *f* 1 dummy; pacifier; comforter; 2 lollipop
sucre *m* **dans le sang** blood sugar level
sueur *f* perspiration; sweat
suffocation *f* suffocation; choking
  ▪ il avait des suffocations = he had fits of choking
sulfamide *m* sulphonamide; sulfonamide
suppositoire *m* suppository
suppuration *f* [AM: formation de pus] suppuration [AM: formation of pus]
suppurer *v* to suppurate
surdité *f* deafness
surdosage *m* overdosage; excess dose
surdose *f* overdose; excess dose
surpoids *m* overweight; excess weight
surveillance *f* **électronique** electronic monitoring
surveillance *f* **médicale** medical supervision
surveillant *m*; **surveillante** *f* head/chief nurse; charge nurse
suture *f* suture
suturer *v* to sew up; to stitch; to suture
sycosis *m* [AM: infection à la zone de la barbe] sycosis [AM: infection of the beard area]
symptomatique *adj* symptomatic
symptôme *m* symptom
synapse *f* synapse
syncope *f* blackout; fainting fit
  ▪ avoir une syncope = to have a blackout/fainting fit
  ▪ tomber en syncope = to blackout; to faint
syndrome *m* syndrome
  ▪ syndrome de Down = Down's syndrome
  ▪ syndrome du choc toxique; SCT = Toxic Shock Syndrome
  ▪ syndrome immunodéficitaire acquis; sida = acquired immunodeficiency syndrome; Aids
  ▪ syndrome prémenstruel; PMS premenstrual tension; PMT
synergie *f* synergy
synergiste *m*; **also** *adj* synergistic
synovial,-e *adj* synovial
synoviale *f* synovial membrane
synovie *f* synovia
  ▪ avoir un épanchement de synovie = to have water on the knee
syphilis *f* syphilis
système *m* system

- système cardio-vasculaire = cardiovascular system
- système digestif = digestive system
- système endocrinien = endocrine system [endocrine glands]
- système immunitaire = immune system
- système lymphatique = lymphatic system
- système nerveux = nervous system
- système parasympathique = parasympathetic nervous system
- système respiratoire = respiratory system

systémique *adj* systemic

T

tabagisme *m* **(syn. nicotinisme)** tobacco addiction; nicotine poisoning (intoxication); tabagism

tableau *m* **d'acuité visuelle** sight testing chart

tache *f* **aveugle** blind spot

tache *f* **café au lait** brown stain/mark on skin

tache *f* **de naissance** birthmark

taches *fpl* **rouges** red spots

tachycardie *f* [AM: acceleration du rythme cardiaque] tachycardia [AM: greatly raised pulse rate]

taie *f* [AM: opacité de la cornée] leukoma; leucoma [AM: corneal opacity]

taille *f* 1 waist; waistline; 2 size

talc *m* talc; talcum powder; baby powder

talon *m* heel

tampon *m* 1 swab (medical); 2 buffer (solution)

tampon *m* **hygiénique** tampon

tamponnement *m* tamponade; tamponage

tapotement *m* tapotement; tapping or percussion massage

tapoter *v* to tap

tarse *m* tarsus
- os du tarse = tarsals

tartre *m* tartar

tassement *m* **de la colonne (vertébrale)** compression of the spinal column

tatouage *m* 1 tattoo; 2 tattooing

taux *m* **de cholestérol du sang** blood cholestrerol level

tégument *m* tegument

teigne *f* ringworm; tinea
teinture *f* 1 tincture; 2 dye; 3 dyeing (eg hair)
- teinture alcoolique = alcoholic tincture
- teinture d'iode = tincture of iodine

téléradiothérapie *f* teleradiotherapy
tempe *f* temple
température *f* temperature
- avoir/faire de la température = to have a temperature
- prendre la température de quelqu'un = to take someone's temperature
- température du sang = blood heat

temps *m* **de coagulation** coagulation time
temps *m* **de latence** latency time
tendon *m* tendon; sinew (muscle tendon)
tendon *m* **d'Achille** Achilles tendon (of heel)
teneur *f* **du sang en alcool éthylique** alcohol content of blood
ténia *m*; **taenia** *m* [AM: ver parasite] tapeworm; taenia [AM: parasitic worm]
tensiomètre *m* [AM: appareil servant à mesurer la pression artérielle]
  sphygmomanometer [AM: instrument measuring blood pressure]
tension *f* **artérielle; tension** *f* blood pressure
- faire de l'hypertension/hypotension = to have high/low blood pressure
- j'ai de la tension/trop de tension = to have high blood pressure/ hypertension
- je souffre d'hypertension = I have high blood pressure
- ma tension est trop élevée/ basse = my blood pressure is too high/ low
- prendre la tension de quelqu'un = to take someone's blood pressure
- sa tension a monté/a baissé = his blood pressure has risen/ has fallen
- tension arteriélle diastolique/systolique diastolic/systolic blood pressure
- tension intraoculaire/oculaire (syn. pression intraoculaire) intraocular pressure
- vérifier la tension = to check the blood pressure

tente *f* **à oxygène** oxygen tent
terme *m* term
- accouchement à terme = full-term delivery
- naître/accoucher avant terme = to be born/delivered prematurely

tertiaire *adj* tertiary
test *m* test
- test d'acuité visuelle = sight test
- test de personnalité = personality test
- test psychologique = psychological test

testicule *m* testicle
- torsion du testicule = torsion of the testicle

testostérone *f* [AM: hormone stéroïde mâle] testosterone [AM: male hormone]
tétanie *f* tetany

tétanos *m* tetanus
- êtes-vous vacciné(e) contre le tétanos? = have you been inoculated against tetanus?

tête *f* head

tétine *f* 1 teat (of baby's bottle); 2 dummy; pacifier

tétracycline *f* [AM: antibiotique]   tetracycline [AM: antibiotic}

thalamus *m* [AM: partie du cerveau]   thalamus [AM: part of brain]

thalassothérapie *f*; **thérapie** *f marine*   thalassotherapy; marine therapy

théâtre *m* **d'opérations**   operating theatre

thérapeutique *f*; **also** *adj*   therapeutics; treatment; therapeutic *(adj)*

thérapie *f*   therapy
- thérapie de groupe = group therapy
- thérapie genique = gene therapy

thermomètre *m*   thermometer
- thermomètre à infrarouges = infrared thermometer
- thermomètre Celsius/centigrade/Fahrenheit = Celsius/centigrade /Fahrenheit thermometer
- thermomètre électronique = electronic thermometer
- thermomètre médical = clinical thermometer

thermothérapie *f*   thermotherapy; heat treatment
- traiter par la thermothérapie = to treat by thermotherapy

thorax *m*   thorax

thrombine *f*   thrombin

thrombose *f*   thrombosis

thrombose *f* **coronarienne**   coronary thrombosis

thymique *adj*   thymic

thymus *m* [AM: glande dont la fonction est de produire des lymphocytes]   thymus [AM: gland involved in lymphocytes production]

thyroïde *f*; **also** *adj*   thyroid; thyroid gland

tibia *m*   shinbone; tibia

tic *m*   tic

tissu *m*   tissue
- tissu conjonctif = connective tissue

toise *f*   height gauge

tolérance *f*   tolerance

tolérer *v*   to tolerate

tomographie *f* [AM: methode radiologique permettant la visualisation des structures anatomique]   tomography [AM: radiological method for sectional scanning of body]

tondeuse *f* **à cheveux**   hair clippers; hair trimmer

tonicité *f*   tone; tonicity; tonus

tonique *m*; **also** *adj*   tonic

tonsille *f* tonsil
tonsillite *f* **(syn. amygdalite)** tonsillitis
topique *adj* topical; local
torsion *f* torsion; twisting
torticolis *m* torticollis; wry neck; stiff neck
toucher *m* sense of touch
  - un toucher rectal/vaginal = rectal/vaginal examination (with fingers)
tourniquet *m* tourniquet
tousser *v* cough (to)
  - toussez = cough
toux *f* cough; coughing
  - elle a une mauvaise toux = she has a bad cough
  - toux de fumeur = smoker's cough
  - toux seche = dry cough
toxémie *f* toxaemia; toxemia
toxicologie *f* toxicology
toxicologue *m,f* toxicologist
toxicomane *m,f* drug addict
toxicomanie *f* drug addiction
toxine *f* toxin
toxique *adj* toxic
toxoplasmose *f* toxoplasmosis
trac *m* stagefright; (exam) nerves
trachée *f* windpipe; trachea
trachéotomie *f* tracheotomy
trachome *m* [AM: infection de l'œil] trachoma [AM: eye infection]
tractus *m* **uvéal (syn. uvée)** uveal tract (eye)
traitement *m* treatment
  - être en traitement = to be having treatment (ie in hospital)
traitement *m* **dentaire** dental treatment
traiter *v* to treat
tranchées *fpl* colic; gripes; tormina; after-pains (of childbirth)
tranquille *adj* calm
tranquillisant,-ante *adj* tranquillizer; tranquillizing
tranquillisant *m* tranquillizer
transfuser *v* transfuse (to)
transfusion *f* transfusion
  - transfusion sanguine; transfusion de sang = blood transfusion
transmettre *v* to transmit; to pass on (eg illness)
transpiration *f* **(syn. sueur)** perspiration; sweat
transplantation *f* transplantation; transplant

100

- transplantation cardiaque/du rein = heart/kidney transplant

transplanter *v* to transplant

trauma *m* trauma

traumatique *adj* traumatic

traumatisme *m* traumatism

travail *m* labour (childbirth)
- entrer en travail = to go into/start labour
- femme en travail = woman in labour
- salle de travail = labour ward

tremblement *m* tremor; trembling; shaking

trembler *v* to tremble; to shake; to shiver

trémor *m* tremor; trembling

trémulation *f* tremor

trépan *m* trepan; trephine

trépanation *f* trepanation; trephination

trépaner *v* to trepan; to trephine

triceps *m* triceps (muscles)

tricostéril *m* sterile compress

trompe *f* **de Fallope** Fallopian tube

tronc *m* trunk

trouble *m* trouble; disorder
- troubles digestifs = digestive disorders
- troubles du langage = speech difficulties
- troubles du sommeil = sleep disorders
- troubles physiologiques = physiological disorders

trousse *f* **à premier secours** first-aid kit

trousse *f* **d'urgence** first aid box

trousse *f* **de premiers soins** first-aid kit

tubage *m* intubation; cannulation

tubaire *adj* tubal

tube *m* **digestif** alimentary canal

tubercule *m* tubercle

tuberculeux,-euse *adj* tuberculous; tubercular
- être tuberculeux = to suffer from tuberculosis

tuberculose *f* tuberculosis

tumeur *f* tumour

tumeur *f* **au/du sein** breast tumour

turista *f* acute attack of diarrhoea

tympan *m* eardrum; tympanum

typhoïde *f*; **fièvre** *f* **typhoïde** typhoid; typhoid fever

typhus *m* typhus

U

ulcération *f* ulceration
ulcère *m* ulcer
- avoir un ulcère à l'estomac = to have a stomach ulcer
- ulcère de l'estomac = peptic ulcer; gastric ulcer
- ulcère gastro-duodénal = peptic ulcer
ulcérer *v* to ulcerate
- blessure qui s'ulcère = wound that ulcerates or festers
- plaie ulcérée = ulcerated wound
ulcéreux,-euse *adj* ulcerous; covered in ulcers
ultraviolet,-ette *adj* ultraviolet
- rayonnement ultraviolet = ultraviolet radiation
- se faire traiter aux rayons ultra-violets = to receive ultraviolet treatment
ultrason *m* ultrasound
ultrasonique *adj* ultrasonic
unité *f* ward (in hospital); unit
- il est à unité 5 = he is in ward 5
- unité de dialyse = dialysis unit
- unité de soins intensifs = intensive care unit
- unité gynécologique = gynaecology unit
- unité ophtalmologique = eye unit; ophthalmology unit
urée *f* urea
uretère *m* ureter
urétral,-e *adj* urethral
urètre *m* urethra
urétrite *f* urethritis
urgence *f* emergency
- je dois aller aux urgences = I need to go to the casualty department
- le service des urgences = the casualty department; casualty
- les urgences = casualty department; A & E (accident and emergency)
- où sont les urgences? = where is casualty?
- une urgence médicale = medical emergency
urgent,-e *adj* urgent
urine *f* urine
urogénital *adj* urogenital
urologie *f* urology
urologue *m,f* urologist
urticaire *f* nettlerash; urticaria; hives
usage *m* use; usage
- à usage externe/interne = for external/internal use

utérus *m* **(syn. matrice)** uterus
- descente f de l'utérus = prolapse of the uterus

uvée *f* **(syn. tractus uvéal)** uveal tract (eye)

V

vaccin *m* vaccine
- vaccin antivariolique = small pox vaccine
- vaccin BCG = BCG vaccine; antituberculosis vaccine
- BCG = bacille de Calmette et Guérin
- vaccin contre la fièvre jaune = yellow fever vaccine
- vaccin contre la rubéole = rubella vaccine

vaccination *f* vaccination

vacciner *v* to vaccinate; to inoculate
- êtes-vous vacciné(e) contre le tétanos? = have you been inoculated against tetanus?
- se faire vacciner = to have a vaccination

vache folle, maladie *f* **de la** mad cow disease

vagal,-e *adj* [AM: qui se rapporte au nerf vague] vagal [AM: relating to vagus nerve]

vagin *m* vagina

vaginal,-e *adj* vaginal
- j'ai une infection vaginale = I have a vaginal infection

vaginite *f* vaginitis

vaisseau *m* **capillaire** capillary

vaisseau *m* **éclaté** burst blood vessel

vaisseau *m* **lymphatique** lymph vessel

vaisseau *m* **sanguin; vaisseaux** *mpl* **sanguins** blood vessel; blood vessels

valériane *f* valerian

valium ® *m* valium ®

valve *f* valve
- valve artificielle = artificial heart valve
- valve cardiaque = heart valve

valvulaire *adj* valvular

valvule *f* valve; valvula
- valvules cardiaques = heart valves

vaporisateur *m*; **vapo** *m* spray; atomizer
- vaporisateur à parfum = perfume atomizer

103

Vaquez, maladie de erythremia
varice *f*; **varices** *fpl* varicose vein; varix
varicelle *f* chickenpox
variole *f* smallpox
vase *m* **de lit** bedpan
vasectomie *f* [AM: résection partielle des canaux déférens] vasectomy [AM: removal of part of the vas deferens]
vaseline ® *f* vaseline ®; petrolatum
vasoconstricteur *m*; **vasoconstricteur,-trice** *adj* vasoconstrictor; vasoconstrictive nerve
vasoconstriction *f* vasoconstriction
vasodilatateur *m*; **vasodilatateur,-trice** *adj* vasodilator; vasodilator nerve
vasodilatation *f* vasodilation
végétalien,-ienne *adj* vegan
végétalisme *m* veganism
végétarien,-ienne *adj* vegetarian
végétarisme *m* vegetarianism
végétations *fpl* **adénoïdes** adenoids
veine *f* vein
  ▪ veine cave inférieure = inferior vena cava
  ▪ veine cave supérieure = superior vena cava
  ▪ veine coronaire = coronary vein
  ▪ veine jugulaire = jugular vein
  ▪ veine porte = portal vein
  ▪ veine pulmonaire = pulmonary vein
veineux,-euse *adj* venous
vélo *m* **d'entrainement; vélo d'appartement** exercise bicycle
vénérien,-ienne *adj* venereal
  ▪ maladies vénériennes = venereal diseases; V.D.
venin *m* venom (eg snake)
ventilation *f* ventilation
  ▪ ventilation respiratoire = respiratory ventilation
ventouse *f* cupping glass; ventouse
ventre *m* abdomen; stomach
  ▪ gonflement du ventre = distension of the stomach
  ▪ j'ai mal au ventre = I have an upset stomach
  ▪ j'ai mal au ventre = I have a pain in my stomach
ventriculaire *adj* ventricular
ventricule *m* ventricle
  ▪ ventricule gauche/droite = left/right ventricle (of heart)
ver *m* **solitaire** tapeworm

verge *f* **(syn. pénis)** penis
vergetures *fpl* stretch marks
vermifuge *m* vermifuge (to remove intestinal worms)
vernis *m* **à ongles** nail varnish; nail polish
verrucide *m* wart remover
verrue *f* wart; verruca
  ▪ verrue plantar = verruca; plantar wart
vertebral,-e *adj* vertebral
vertèbre *f* vertebra (vertebrae *pl*)
  ▪ vertèbres cervicales = cervical vertebrae
  ▪ vertèbres dorsales = dorsal vertebrae
  ▪ vertèbres lombaires = lumbar vertebrae
vertébré *m* vertebrate
vertige *m* dizziness; vertigo; giddiness
  ▪ avoir des vertiges = to suffer from vertigo
  ▪ j'ai des vertiges = I feel dizzy
vertigineux,-euse *adj* vertiginous
vésicatoire *m*; also *adj* vesicatory
vésicule *f* vesicle; blister
  ▪ vésicule biliaire = gall bladder
  ▪ vésicules génitales = genital warts
vessie *f* bladder; urinary bladder
vibrations *fpl* vibrations; vibromassage
  ▪ traitement par vibrations = vibromassage
vieillesse *f* old age
vieillissement *m* ageing
  ▪ retarder le vieillissement = to slow down the ageing process
vignette *f* detachable label on medicines for reimbursement by social security
viol *m* rape
violer *v* to rape
virilisation *f* virilism
virologie *f* virology
virus *m* virus
virus de l'immunodéficience humaine [AM: virus responsable du sida] human
  immunodeficiency virus; HIV [AM: virus causing aids]
visage *m* face
viscéral,-e *adj* visceral
viscères *mpl* viscera
vision *f* eyesight; vision
vision *f* **double** double vision
vitaliseur *m* vitaliser

105

vitalité *f* vitality
vitamine *f* vitamin
- comprimé *m* de vitamines = vitamin tablet/pill
- vitaminé = with added vitamins; vitamin enriched
- vitamine C = vitamin C

voie *f* duct; pathway; tract
- voies biliaires = biliary ducts
- voies lacrymales = tear ducts
- voies urinaires = urinary tract

voile *m* au poumon   shadow on the lung
voiture *f* d'invalide   invalid carriage
volémie *f* blood volume
volvulus *m*   [AM: torsion de l'intestin provoquant un occlusion]   volvulus   [AM: twisting of intestine causing blockage]
vomi *m*   vomit
vomir *v*   to vomit
vomissement *m*   vomiting; vomit
- être pris de vomissements = to start to vomit
- j'ai eu des vomissements = I have been vomiting

voûte *f* crânienne (syn. calotte crânienne)   dome of the skull; calvaria
voûte *f* palatine; **voûte** *f* du palais   roof of the mouth; bony palate
voûte *f* plantaire   longitudinal arch of the foot
vue *f*   eyesight; vision
vulve *f*   vulva
vulvite *f*   vulvitis

W, Y, Z

wheezing *m*   wheezing
yeux *mpl*   eyes
yoga *m*   yoga
zona *m*   (syn. herpés zoster)   shingles; herpes zoster
zygote *m*   zygote

A

abasia [AM: motor incoordination in walking] abasie *f* [AM: incapacité de marcher par trouble de la coordination des mouvements]

abatement (eg of pain) rémission *f*

abscess abcès *m*
- gumboil = abcès à la gencive
- I have an abscess = j'ai un abcès
- to drain an abscess = vider un abcès

abdomen abdomen *m*; ventre *m*

abdominal abdominal,-e adj

abdominal cavity cavité *f* abdominale

abduction abduction *f*

aberration aberration *f*

aberration, spherical aberration *f* sphérique

abnormality difformité *f*, malformation *f*

abort (to) avorter *v*
- to abort = faire avorter

abortion avortement *m*; interruption *f* (volontaire) de grossesse; IVG
- to have an abortion = se faire avorter

abrasion écorchure *f*; érosion *f* (syn. exulcération)

absorption absorption *f*

acarid; tick; mite acarien *m*

accident accident *m*

acetyl salicylic acid (aspirin) acide *m* acétylsalicylique

ache; pain douleur *f*
- a constant pain = une douleur persistante
- a dull ache = une douleur sourde
- a nagging pain = une douleur irritante
- an intermittent pain = une douleur intermittente
- a sharp pain = une douleur aiguë
- a throbbing pain = une douleur irritante
- what kind of pain is it ? = quelle genre de douleur éprouver vous?

aches and pains; weakness courbatures *fpl*
- I am feeling weak; I have aches and pains = j'ai des courbatures
- to be stiff = avoir des courbatures

Achilles tendon (of heel) tendon *m* d'Achille

acidity acidité *f*

acidosis acidose *f*

acne acné *f*

acne (spot) bouton *m* d'acné

acne rosacea   acné *f* rosacée; rosacée; couperose *f*
acne, cream, gel etc. for treatment of   antiacnéique *m*
acoumetry   [AM: evaluation of hearing]   acoumétrie *f* [AM: evaluation de l'acuité auditive]
acquired   acquis,-ise *adj*
- acquired character = caractère acquis
- acquired immunity = immunité acquise
acromegaly   [AM: rare disease causing enlargement of hands, face etc.]   acromégalie *f* [AM: maladie rare, provoquant augmentation des mains, de la tête etc]
activated charcoal; activated carbon   charbon *m* activé
acuity; acuteness   acuité *f*
acupuncture   acupuncture *f*
acute; sharp   aigu, aiguë *adj*
- acute respiratory disease = maladie aigüe de l'appareil respiratoire
- sharp pain = une douleur aiguë
Adam's apple   pomme *f* d'Adam
addiction (to a drug)   dépendance *f*
Addison's disease   maladie *f* d'Addison; maladie *f* bronzée
adduction   adduction *f*
adenitis   [AM: inflammation of a lymphatic ganglion]   adénite *f* [AM: inflammation d'un ganglion lymphatique]
adenoids   végétations *fpl* adénoïdes
adenoma   [AM: benign tumour on a gland]   adénome *m* [AM: tumeur bénigne sur une glande]
adhesion   adhérence *f*
adhesive plaster   pansement *m* adhésif
adhesive tape   ruban *m* de tissu adhésif
adhesive tape (medical); sticking plaster   sparadrap *m*
- microporous adhesive tape = sparadrap micro-poreux
adolescence   adolescence *f*
adolescent   adolescent,-e *adj*
adolescent   adolescent *m*; adolescente *f*
adrenal gland; suprarenal gland   glande *f* surrénale; surrénale *f*
adrenaline; epinephrine   adrénaline *f*
adult   adulte *m,f*
advise (to); recommend (to)   conseiller *v*
aerobics   aérobic *m*
aerocoly   aérocolie *f*
aerogastria   aérogastrie *f*
aerophagy   aérophagie
aerosol   aérosol *m*
affect (to); reach (to)   atteindre *v*
affected   atteint,-e *adj*

- to be suffering from an illness = être atteint d'une maladie

affection maladie *f*; affection *f*

after-sun lotion lotion *f* après-soleil

aftercare (eg convalescent care) post-cure *f*

aftershave aftershave *m*; lotion *f* après-rasage

ageing vieillissement *m*
- to slow down the ageng process = retarder le vieillissement

ageing (prevention of) anti-âge *adj* (prévention)

agglutinate (to) agglutiner *v*

agglutination; clumping agglutination *f*

agglutinin agglutinine *f*

AIDS; aids; acquired immune deficiency syndrome SIDA; sida; syndrome immunodéficitaire acquis

albinism albinisme *m*

albumin albumine *f*

albuminuria albuminurie *f*

alcohol alcool *m*
- pure alcohol; absolute alcohol = alcool absolu
- surgical spirit = alcool à 90 (degrés); alcool modifié à 90

alcohol content of blood teneur *f* du sang en alcool éthylique

alcoholism alcoolisme *m*

alimentary canal tube *m* digestif

alkaloid alcaloïde *m*

allergen allergène *m*

allergic allergique *adj* (à)
- I am allergic to penicillin = je suis allergique à la pénicilline

allergy allergie *f*
- allergy alleviating = antiallergique *adj*
- contact allergy = allergie de contact
- respiratory allergy = allergie respiratoire
- skin allergy = allergie cutanée

allopathy [AM: therapeutic method] allopathie *f* [AM: méthode thérapeutique]

alopecia [AM: hair loss] alopécie *f* [AM: chute des cheveux]

alopecia areata [AM: hair loss in patches] pelade *f* [AM: chute des cheveux en plaques]

alpha-blocker; alpha-blocking alphabloquant *m*

alveolitis (of the lungs) alvéolite *f* pulmonaire

Alzheimer's disease [AM: degeneration of the brain cortex] maladie *f* d'Alzheimer
[AM: dégénérescence cérébrale]

ambulance ambulance *f*

ambulance service service *m* ambulancier

ambulatory ambulatoire *adj*

111

androsterone

- ambulatory care = traitement ambulatoire
- ambulatory patient = malade ambulatoire

amenorrhoea [AM: absence of menstruation] aménorrhée *f* [AM: absence des règles]

ammonia ammoniaque *f*

amnesia amnésie *f*

amniocentesis amniocentèse *f*

amniotic amniotique adj
- amniotic cavity = cavité *f* amniotique
- amniotic fluid = liquide *m* amniotique
- amniotic sac = poche *f* des eaux

amoeba; ameba [AM: parasitic bacterium] amibe *f* {AM: parasite bactérien]

amount; proportion; quantity determination; dosage (eg medicine) dosage *m*

amphetamine amphétamine *f*

ampoule; phial ampoule *f*

ampulla ampoule *f*
- rectal ampulla = ampoule rectale

amputation amputation *f*

anabolic steroid anabolisant *m* stéroïdien; anabolisant *m*; also adj

anaemia anémie *f*
- pernicious anaemia = anémie pernicieuse
- pernicious anaemia = anémie/maladie de Biermer
- pernicious anaemia = anémie pernicieuse progressive

anaemic anémique adj

anaesthetic; anesthesic anesthésique *m*; also adj
- agent anesthésique = anaesthetic

anal anal,-e adj

anal canal; rectum canal *m* anal

anal cleft raie *f* des fesses

anal sphincter sphincter *m* anal

analgesia analgésie *f*

analgesic; painkiller; anodyne analgésique *m*

analysis analyse *f*

anaphylactic anaphylactique adj
- anaphylactic shock = choc anaphylactique

anaphylaxy; anaphylaxis anaphylaxie *f*

anasarca [AM: general oedema of the tissues] anasarque *f* [AM: œdème généralisé du tissu]

anatomical anatomique adj

anatomy anatomie *f*

androgen (male hormone) androgène *m*

androsterone (male hormone) androstérone *f*

112

anesthesia; anaesthesia anesthésie *f*
- epidural anesthesia = anesthésie épidurale
- general anesthesia = anesthésie générale
- local anesthesia = anesthésie locale
- peridural anesthesia = anesthésie péridurale
- to give someone a local/general anaesthetic = faire une anesthésie locale/générale

anesthetist; anaesthetist anesthésiste *m,f*

anesthetize (to); anaesthetize (to); block (to) (pain) anesthésier *v*

aneurism; aneurysm anévrisme *m*
- arterial aneurism = anévrisme artériel

angeitis angéite *f*

anger; fit; tantrum colère *f*

angina pectoris angine *f* de poitrine; angor *m*; crampe *f* de poitrine

angiocardiography [AM: x-ray examination of heart] angiocardiographie *f* [AM: examen aux rayons X du cœur]

angiography angiographie *f*

angioma [AM: tumour composed of blood vessels] angiome *m* [AM: tumeur formée par agglomération de vaisseaux sanguins]

angioneurotic oedema [AM: severe allergic hives] œdème *m* de Quinke [AM: réaction allergique, comme l'urticaire]

angor angoisse *f*

ankle cheville *f*
- I have twisted my ankle = je me suis tordu la cheville

ankylosing spondylitis spondylarthrite *f* ankylosante

ankylosis [AM: part or total immobility of a joint] ankylose *f* [AM: limitation de la mobilité d'une articulation]

ankylostomiasis; hookworm disease ankylostomiase *f*, ankylostomose *f*

anomalous anormal *adj*; irrégulier *adj*

anorexia anorexie f

anorexia nervosa anorexie *f* mentale

antacid antiacide *m*; also *adj*

anthelmintic; antihelminthic [AM: remedy for eliminating intestinal worms] antihelminthique *m*, also *adj* [AM: médicament pour l'élimination des vers intestinaux]

anthrax anthrax *m*; charbon *m*

anti- (blood) platelet aggregation antiagrégant plaquettaire

anti-inflammatory anti-inflammatoire *adj*

antiacne cream/lotion produit contre l'acné

antiarthritique *m*; also *adj* drug/treatment alleviating arthritis

antiasthmatique *m*; also *adj* drug/treatment alleviating asthma

antibacterial antibactérien,-ienne *adj*

antibiotic antibotique *m*; also *adj*

apoplexy

- to be on antibiotics = être sous antibiotiques
antibiotic ointment   pommade *f* antibiotique
antibody   anticorps *m*
anticancer (eg treatment)   anticancéreux,-euse *adj*
  - cancer hospital = centre anticancéreux
  - cancer serum = sérum anticancéreux
anticoagulant   anticoagulant *m*; also *adj*
antidepressant   antidépresseur *m*; antidépressif *m*; also *adj*
antidiuretic   antidiurétique *m*; also *adj*
antidote   antidote *m*; contrepoison *m*
antifungal   antifongique *m*; also *adj*
antigen   antigène *m*
antigenic   antigénique *adj*
antihistamine   antihistaminique *m*; also *adj*
  - antihistamine = produit *m* antihistaminique
antineoplastic   anticancéreux,-euse *adj*
antioxidant   antioxydant *m*; also *adj*
antipyretic   antipyrétique *m*; also *adj*
antiscorbutic   antiscorbutique *adj*
antisepsis   antisepsie *f*
antiseptic   antiseptique *m*; also *adj*
antispasmodic (eg drug)   antispasmodique *m*; also *adj*
antitoxic   antitoxique *adj*
antitoxin   antitoxine *f*
antitussive   antitussif *m*; antitussif,-ive *adj*
antiviral   antiviral,-e *adj*
antiwrinkle cream   crème *f* antirides
antiwrinkle face-pack   masque *m* antirides
anuresis; anuria   anurèse *f*
anuria; anuresis   anurie *f*
anus   anus *m*
anxiety   anxiété *f*; angoisse *f*
aorta   aorte *f*
aphasia [AM: inability to speak due to brain disease or injury]   aphasie *f* [AM: incapacité de parler qui est due à une atteinte cérébrale]
aphonia [AM: loss of voice]   aphonie *f* [AM: extinction de voix]
aphrodisiac   aphrodisiaque *m*
apophysis; process [AM: bony outgrowth   apophyse *f* [AM: saillie osseuse]
apoplectic   apoplectique *adj*
apoplexy; stroke   apoplexie *f*
  - apoplectic fit ; to have a stroke = attaque *f* d'apoplexie

114

appendectomy; appendicectomy [AM: removal of appendix] **appendicectomie** *f* [AM: ablation de l'appendice]
appendicitis appendicite *f*
- acute appendicitis = appendicite aiguë
appendix appendice *m*
appetite appétit *m*
- appetite depressant = coupe-faim *m inv*
- to lose one's appetite = perdre l'appétit
apply (to) (eg ointment, dressing) appliquer *v*; mettre *v*
arch of the foot, longitudinal voûte plantaire
arm bras *m*
- my arm is broken = mon bras est cassé
armpit; axilla aisselle *f*
aromatherapy aromathérapie *f*
arteriosclerosis artériosclérose *f*
artery artère *f*
- carotid artery = artère *f* carotide
- cubital artery = artère *f* cubitale
- facial artery = artère *f* faciale
- femoral artery = artère *f* fémorale
- humeral artery = artère *f* humérale
- pulmonary artery = artère *f* pulmonaire
- radial artery = artère *f* radiale
- subclavian artery = artère *f* sous-clavière
- tibial artery = artère *f* tibiale
arthritis arthrite *f*
arthritis; osteoarthritis arthrite *f* sèche déformante; arthrite chronique dégénér-ative; arthrose
artificial heart valve prothèse *f* valvulaire; valve *f* artificielle
artificial insemination by donor; AID insémination *f* artificielle avec donneur; IAD
artificial teeth dents *mpl* artificiels
asbestosis asbestose *f*
ascites ascite *f*
ascorbic acid (vitamin C) acide *m* ascorbique
Asian flu grippe *f* asiatique
asphyxia asphyxie *f*
asphyxiation; suffocation; choking; breathlessness étouffement *m*
- feeling of suffocation or breathlessness = sensation d'étouffement
- to die of suffocation = mourir d'étouffement
- to have fits of breathlessness = avoir des étouffements
aspirin aspirine *f*

- aspirin tablet = comprimé *m* d'aspirine
- I am allergic to aspirin = je suis allergique à l'aspirine
- soluble aspirin = aspirine soluble

asthenia [AM: diminution of strength; debility]   asthénie *f* [AM: diminution des forces; débilité]

asthenic   asthénique *adj*

asthma   asthme *m*

asthmatic   asthmatique *adj*
- I am asthmatic = je suis asthmatique

astigmatism (of eye)   astigmatisme *m*

astragalus; talus, anklebone   astragale *m*

astringent   astringent *m*; also *adj*
- astringent lotion = lotion astringente

ataxia; ataxy   ataxie *f*
- locomotor ataxia = ataxie locomotrice

atrium   l'oreillette *f* du cœur

atrophy [AM: loss in weight or volume of an organ]   atrophie *f* [AM: diminution de poids ou de volume d'un organe]

atrophy (to)   atrophier *v*

atropine   atropine *f*

attack; fit; crisis   crise *f*
- appendicitis = crise d'appendicite
- asthma attack = crise d'asthme
- bilious or liverish attack = crise de foie
- coughing attack/fit = crise de toux
- epileptic fit = crise d'épilepsie
- heart attack = crise cardiaque
- to throw a tantrum; to throw a fit = piquer/faire une crise

audiogram   audiogram *m*

audiometer   audiomètre *m*

audiometry [AM: instrumental measurement of hearing]   audiométrie *f* [AM: mesure instrumentale de l'audition]

auricle; external ear   pavillon *m* auriculaire; pavillon *m* de l'oreille

auricle (heart); atrium   oreillette *f*; l'oreillette du cœur
- left auricle = oreillette *f* gauche
- right auricle = oreillette *f* droite

auricular (ear, heart)   auriculaire *adj*

autism   autisme *m*

autistic   autiste *adj*; autistique *adj*

autistic person   autiste *m,f*

auto-immunity   auto-immunité *f*

auto-intoxication   auto-intoxication *f* (syn. autotoxicose; autotoxémie)

autoclave [AM: appliance used for steam sterilization] autoclave *m* [AM: appareil utilisé pour la stérilisation par la vapeur]
autogenous; autogenic autogène *adj*
autolysis autolyse *f*
automatism automatisme *m*
autoplasty autoplastie *f*
autopsy autopsie *f*
autosuggestion autosuggestion *f*
autotoxin autotoxine *f*
awareness; consciousness; conscience conscience *f*
  ▪ to lose/regain consciousness = perdre/reprendre conscience
axilla aisselle *f*

B

baby bébé *m*
  ▪ to be expecting a baby = attendre un bébé
baby food aliments pour bébés; alimentation *f* pour bébé
baby lotion lait *m* de toilette pour bébés
baby powder talc *m*
baby shampoo shampooing *m* pour bébés
baby wipes lingettes *fpl*
baby's bib bavoir *m*
baby's bottle biberon *m*
  ▪ to bottle feed = nourir au biberon
bacillus bacille *m*
  ▪ *Escherichia coli* = colibacille *m*
back dos *m*
  ▪ backache = mal de dos
  ▪ I have pain in my back = j'ai mal dans le dos
  ▪ small of the back = chute *f* des reins
back of the knee jarret *m*
back pain mal *m* de dos; maux *mpl* de dos
back teeth dents *fpl* de derrière; dents du fond
backache mal *m* aux reins; mal de reins
bacterial bactérien,-ienne *adj*
bactericide bactéricide *m*; also *adj*
bacteriological bactériologique *adj*

bacteriologist bactériologiste *m,f*
bacteriology bactériologie *f*
bacterium; bacteria (*pl*) bactérie *f*; bactéries *fpl*
bad tooth dent *f* gâtée
- decayed tooth = carie dentaire
balanitis [AM: inflammation of the glans penis] balanite *f* [AM: inflammation du gland de la verge]
bald chauve *adj*
baldness calvitie *f*
bandage bande *f*
- elastique bandage = bande elastique
- plaster bandage = bande plâtrée
bandage (prepared dressing) bandage *m*
- to bandage someone up = faire un bandage à quelqu'un
bandage (to) bander *v*
bandage, gauze roller bande *f* de gaze
bandage, triangular bandage *m* triangulaire
bank banque *f*
- blood bank = banque de sang
- plasma bank = banque de plasma
- skin bank = banque de peau
- sperm bank = banque de sperme
barbiturate barbiturique *m*
bare (to); strip (to) dénuder *v*
- to strip off = se dénuder
barium meal (prior to x-ray) bouillie *f* de sulfate de baryum
bath salts sels *mpl* de bain
BCG vaccine; antituberculosis vaccine vaccin *m* BCG
- BCG = bacille de Calmette et Guérin
bed lit *m*
- private bed (in hospital) = lit privé
- to stay in bed = rester au lit
bedpan bassin *m* (hygiénique); bassin *m* de lit; vase *m* de lit
bedsore escarre *f*
bedwetting incontinence *f* nocturne
belladonna belladone *f*
benign bénin, bénigne *adj* (ant. malin, maligne)
- benign tumour = tumeur bénigne
beta-blocker; beta-blocking bêtabloquant m; bêtabloqueur *m*
better meilleur; mieux *adj*
- he got better very quickly after his illness = il s'est très vite remis de sa maladie

- he is much better now = il va/se porte bien mieux maintenant
biceps biceps *m*
bile bile *f*
bile duct canal *m* biliaire
bilharzia; bilharziasis [AM: infestation by worms (bilharzia)] bilharziose *f* (syn.
  schistosomiase) [AM: infestation par vers (bilharzies)]
biliary colic colique *f* biliaire
biliary ducts voies *fpl* biliaires
bilious bilieux,-ieuse *adj*
biliousness affection *f* hépatique
bilirubin bilirubine *f*
biliverdin biliverdine *f*
bind (to) (eg artery) ligaturer v
biochemical laboratory laboratoire *m* biochimique
biochemistry biochimie *f*
biodegradability biodégradabilité *f*
biodegradable biodégradable *adj*
biology biologie *f*
biopsy biopsie *f*
biorhythm biorythme *m*
birth control; family planning contrôle *m* des naissances (syn. planification
  familiale)
birthmark tache *f* de naissance
bite morsure *f*
- a dog bite = une morsure (de) chien
- a snake bite = une morsure (de) serpent
black eye œil *m* poché; œil au beurre noir
blackhead; comedo comédon *m*
blackout (faint) évanouissement *m*
blackout; fainting fit syncope *f*
- to have a blackout/fainting fit = avoir une syncope
- to blackout; to faint = tomber en syncope
bladder, gall vésicule *f* biliaire
bladder; urinary bladder vessie *f*
bleach, household (liquid) eau *f* de Javel
bleed (to) saigner v
bleeding saignement *f*
bleeding; blood letting saignée *f*
blepharitis [AM: inflammation of the eyelids] blépharite *f* [AM: inflammation des
  paupières]
blind man/woman aveugle *m,f*

119

blood pressure

blind spot   point *m* aveugle; tache *f* aveugle
blindness   cécité *f*
blister (to)   se couvrir d'ampoules *v*
   ▪ couvert d'ampoules = blistered
blister   ampoule *f*
   ▪ blister plaster = pansement pour l'ampoule
blister pack (for pills etc)   plaquette *f*
bloating; distension (of stomach)   ballonnement m
block   bloc m
   ▪ cardiac block = bloc cardiaque; bloc auriculo-ventriculaire
   ▪ operating suite = bloc opératoire
blockage, intestinal   occlusion *f*
blockage; blocking   blocage *m*
blood   sang *m*
blood bank   banque *f* de sang
blood cell   cellule *f* sanguine
blood cell, red/white   globule *m* rouge/blanc
blood corpuscle; blood cell   globule *m* sanguin
blood cholesterol   taux *m* de cholestérol du sang
blood clot   caillot *m* de sang
blood clotting agent   agent *m* coagulant du sang
blood compatibility   compatibilité *f* sanguine
blood count   numération *f* globulaire
blood donation   don *m* du sang
blood group; blood type   groupe *m* sanguin
   ▪ my blood group is (A, B, AB, O) = mon groupe sanguin est (A, B, AB, O)
blood grouping   recherche *f* du groupe sanguin
blood heat   température *f* du sang
blood plasma   plasma *m* sanguin
blood platelets   plaquettes *fpl* sanguines
blood poisoning   empoisonnement *m* du sang
blood pressure   tension *f* artérielle
   ▪ his blood pressure has risen/has fallen = sa tension a monté/a baissé
   ▪ I have high blood pressure = je souffre d'hypertension
   ▪ I have high blood pressure/ hypertension = j'ai de la tension; j'ai trop de tension
   ▪ my blood pressure is too high/ low = ma tension est trop élevée/ basse
   ▪ to check blood pressure = verifier la tension
   ▪ to have high/low blood pressure = faire de l'hypertension/hypotension
   ▪ to take someone's blood pressure = prendre la tension de quelqu'un
blood pressure, diastolic/systolic   pression *f* (artérielle) diastolique/systolique;
   tension *f* arteriélle diastolique/systolique

120

blood sample; taking a blood sample prise *f* de sang
blood sugar level sucre *m* dans le sang
blood test; blood examination analyse *f* de sang; examen *m* du sang
blood transfusion transfusion *f* sanguine; transfusion de sang
blood vessel; blood vessels vaisseau *m* sanguin; vaisseaux mpl sanguins
blood volume volémie *f*
blood, contaminated sang *m* contaminé
bloodletting saignée *f*
bloodshot (eyes) injecté (de sang)
blow (to); insufflate (to) insuffler *v*
blusher (cosmet) blush *m*
body corps *m*
 ▪ foreign body = corps étranger
 ▪ the medical profession = le corps médical
 ▪ vitreous body (eye) = corps vitré
 ▪ yellow body, corpus luteum = corps jaune
body lotion lait *m* pour le corps
boil; furuncle furoncle m; clou *m*
bolus; pellet bol *m*
bone os *m*
bone; bony osseux,-euse *adj*
booster (vaccination); booster shot; booster dose piqûre *f* de rappel; rappel *m*
boric acid acide *m* borique
bottle, small; phial flacon *m*
 ▪ small bottle with dropper = flacon doseur
bottle feeding allaitement *m* artificiel
bottle warmer (baby's bottle) chauffe-biberon *m*
botulism [AM: food poisoning due to toxin of the bacillus C.botulinum] botulisme *m* [AM: intoxication alimentaire provoquée par le bacille C.botulinum]
brace appareil *m* orthopédique
brace(s) (for teeth) appareil *m* dentaire; appareil orthodontique
brain cerveau *m*
brain damage lésions *fpl* cérébrales
brain fever fièvre *f* cérébrale
break (to) casser *v*
 ▪ broken = cassé
 ▪ to break one's rib = se casser une côte
breakdown; exhaustion coup *m* de pompe
breaking; crushing enfoncement *m*
 ▪ he has a fractured skull = il souffre d'un enfoncement de la boîte crânienne
 ▪ he has crushed ribs = il souffre d'un enfoncement de la cage thoracique

breast sein *m*
- abscess of the breast = abcès du sein
- breast cancer = cancer du sein
- breast tumeur = tumeur *f* au/du sein

breast-feeding allaitement *m* maternel

breastfeed (to) allaiter v
- I'm breastfeeding = j'allaite mon enfant
- to bottle feed = allaiter au biberon

breath; breathing haleine *f*
- bad breath = mauvaise haleine

Breathalyser (instrument) Alcootest ® *m*
- to breathalyse = faire subir l'Alcootest à

breathalyzer test alcootest m

breathe (to) respirer *v*
- breathe in = respirez!
- I have difficulties in breathing = j'ai de la peine à respirer
- take a deep breath = respirez bien fort
- to have difficulty breathing = respirer avec difficulté

breathing; respiration respiration *f*
- artificial respiration = respiration artificielle
- assisted *v*entilation = respiration assistée

breech birth; breech delivery accouchement *m* par le siège; siège *m*

bring down (eg a fever) calmer *v*

bronchial bronchique *adj*

bronchiole bronchiole *f*

bronchitis bronchite *f*

bronchodilator bronchodilatateur *m*

bronchopneumonia broncho-pneumonie *f*

bronchus, right/left bronche *f* droite/gauche

brown stain/mark on skin tache *f* café au lait

brucellosis; undulant fever; Malta fever brucellose *f*

bruise bleu *m*; contusion *f*; ecchymose *f*; meurtrissure *f*
- body covered with bruises = corps couvert d'ecchymoses/ de meurtrissures

bruise; haematoma hématoma *m*

bruise (to) faire *v* un bleu à; contusionner *v*; meurtrir *v*
- a bruised arm/knee = un bras/un genou contussioné
- brused eye/cheek/ribs/back/muscle = un œil meurtri/une joue meurtrie/des côtes meurtries/un dos meurtri/un muscle meurtri
- to bruise one's arm = se meurtrir le bras
- to bruise one's foot = se faire un bleu au pied

bruxism (grinding of teeth) mâchonnement *m*

122

buccal; mouth buccal,-e *adj*
buffer (solution) tampon *m*
bulimia; bulimia nervosa boulimie *f*
bump bosse *f*
bunion oignon *m*
burn brûlure *f*
  ▪ first/second/third degree burn = brûlure du premier/deuxième/troisième degré
bursa bourse *f* séreuse; bourse *f* synoviale
bursitis bursite *f*; hygroma *m*
burst blood vessel vaisseau *m* éclaté
buttock fesse *f*
  ▪ the buttocks; the bottom = les fesses
buttock; gluteal fessier,-ière *adj*
  ▪ gluteal muscles = muscles fessiers
bypass; bypass operation pontage *m*
  ▪ coronary bypass = pontage coronarien
  ▪ heart bypass operation = pontage cardiaque

C

caecum [AM: part of large intestine] caecum *m* [AM: partie de gros intestin]
Caesarean (section) [AM: incision allowing delivery of baby from the uterus] césarienne *f*
  [AM: incision permettant d'extraire un nouveau-né de l'utérus]
  ▪ she had a Caesarean = elle a eu une césarienne
.**calamine** calamine *f*
  ▪ calamine lotion = lotion calmante à la calamine
calcaneum [AM: bone of heel] calcanéum *m* [AM: os de talon]
calcification calcification *f*
calcium calcium *m*
calculous pierreux,-euse *adj*
calculus; stone (eg in bladder, gall bladder) calcul *m*
calf mollet *m*
callus cal *m*; durillon *m*; callosité *f*
calm down (to) calmer *v*
calmative; sedative calmant *m*
calorie (heat unit) calorie *f*
cancer cancer *m*
  ▪ breast cancer = cancer du sein

- cancer of the oesophagus = cancer de l'œsophage
- cancer of the stomach = cancer de l'estomac
- cervical cancer = cancer du col de l'utérus
- lung cancer = cancer du poumon
- renal cancer = cancer du rein
- skin cancer = cancer de la peau

cancer patient cancéreux m, cancéreuse f
cancer specialist cancérologue m,f
cancer ward service m de cancer
cancerous; malignant cancéreux,-euse adj
Candida albicans (a fungus) Candida albicans
candidosis; candidiasis; moniliasis candidose f, moniliase f
canine (tooth); eye tooth canine f
cannabis cannabis m
capacity capacité f
capillary vaisseau m capillaire
capsule capsule f
carbon monoxide oxyde de carbone m; monoxyde de carbone m
carcinogen; cancer-causing; carcinogenic cancérigène m; cancérogène m;
  also adj; carcinogène m; also adj
carcinoma carcinome m
cardiac cardiaque adj

- I have heart trouble = je suis cardiaque
- to suffer/ to have a heart condition = être cardiaque

cardiac arrest arrêt cardiaque
cardiac murmur; heart murmur souffle m cardiaque; souffle m au cœur
cardiac plexus plexus m cardiaque
cardiogram cardiogramme m
cardiograph cardiographe m
cardiography cardiographie f
cardiologist cardiologue m,f
cardiology cardiologie f
cardiovascular cardio-vasculaire adj

- cardiovascular accident = accident cardio-vasculaire
- cardiovascular disease = maladie f cardio-vasculaire
- cardiovascular system = système m cardio-vasculaire

carditis cardite f
caries carie f

- dental caries = carie dentaire

carotene carotène m
carotid [AM: carotid arteries of the neck and head] carotide f [AM: artères corotides du cou

124

et de la tête]

carotid carotidien *adj*

carpal canal canal *m* carpien

carpals [AM: wrist bones] carpes *mpl*; os du carpe *mpl* [AM: les os du poignet]

carpus carpe *m*

carrier porteur *m,f*
- germ carrier = porteur de germes

cartilage cartilage *m*

case cas *m*

castration castration *f*

casualty department; A & E (accident and emergency) les urgences
- I need to go to the casualty department = je dois aller aux urgences
- the casualty department = le service des urgences
- where is casualty? = où sont les urgences?

catalepsy catalepsie *f*

cataract cataracte *f*
- he has been operated on for a cataract = il a été opéré de la cataracte

catarrh catarrhe *m*; rhume *m* (chronique)
- to have catarrh = avoir des glaires

catarrhal catarrhal,-e *adj*

catgut catgut *m*

cathartic cathartique *m*; also *adj*

catheter cathéter *m*; sonde *f*
- catheter = sonde à canal central
- catheter = sonde creuse
- feeding tube = sonde d'alimentation
- stomach tube = sonde gastrique
- to put a catheter in someone = mettre une sonde à quelqu'un
- urethral catheter = sonde urétrale

catheterization cathétérisme *m*; sondage *m*

catheterize (to) sonder *v*

cauterization cautérisation *f*

cauterize (to) cautériser *v*

cavernous; hollow caverneux,-euse *adj*
- lung with cavitations; lung with cavernous lesion = poumon caverneux

cavity cavité *f*

cell cellule *f*

cellulitis cellulite *f*

cerebellum cervelet *m*

cerebral cérébral,-e *adj*

cerebrospinal cérébro-spinal,-e *adj*

cerebrum; brain cerveau *m*
cerumen; earwax cérumen *m*
cervix of uterus col *m* de l'utérus; col utérin
chalazion [AM: small cyst in or on eyelid] chalazion *m* [AM: petite nodule dans la paupière]
chancre chancre *m*
  ▪ chancre = chancre syphilitique
  ▪ chancroid; soft chancre = chancre mou; chancrelle *f*
chap (to) (eg skin) crevasser *v*
  ▪ to become chapped = se crevasser
chapping gerçure *f*
  ▪ to have badly chapped hands = avoir les mains pleines de gerçures
cheek joue *f*
cheekbone pommette *f*
chemist's; pharmacy pharmacie *f*
  ▪ night pharmacy; pharmacy in service; pharmacy that's open = pharmacie de
  garde
chemotherapy chimiotherapie *f*
chest; breasts poitrine *f*
  ▪ I have a pain in my chest = je ressens une douleur dans la poitrine
chickenpox varicelle *f*
chilblain engelure *f*
  ▪ I have a chilblain on my foot = j'ai une engelure à mon pied
child enfant *m,f*
  ▪ blue baby = enfant bleu
child's chamber pot; potty pot *m* (d'enfant)
childbirth; delivery accouchement *m*
  ▪ a difficult/an easy birth/delivery = accouchement difficile/facile
  ▪ full term/premature birth = accouchement à terme/ avant terme
  ▪ induced delivery = accouchement provoqué
chill refroidissement *m*; coup *m* de froid
  ▪ to catch a chill = prendre un refroidissement
chill (shiver) frisson *m*
  ▪ I am shivery = j'ai des frissons
chin menton *m*
chin bandage mentonnière *f*
chiropodist; podiatrist (US) pédicure *m,f*
chiropody; podiatry (US) soins *mpl* du pédicure; soins *mpl* du pied; podologie *f*
chiropractic chiropractie *f*; chiropraxie *f*
chiropractor chiropracteur *m*
Chlamydia Chlamydiae *f*
chloasma (skin pigmentation) masque *m* de grossesse

chloral hydrate   hydrate *m* de chloral
cholera   choléra *m*
cholesterol   cholestérol *m*
chorea; St. Vitus' dance   chorée *f*
- Huntingdon's chorea = chorée de Huntingdon
choroid   [AM: eyeball membrane]   choroïde *f* [AM: membrane du globe oculaire]
choroiditis   [AM: inflammation of the choroid]   choroidite *f* [AM: inflammation de la choroïde]
chromosome   chromosome *m*
- X or Y chromosome = chromosome X ou Y
chromosomic aberration   aberration *f* chromosomique
chronic   chronique *adj*
chronic disease   maladie *f* chronique
chronic lupus erythematosis   lupus *m* érythémateux chronique
chyle   chyle *m*
circulation   circulation *f*
- circulation of blood = circulation sanguine
circumcision   circoncision *f*
cirrhosis   cirrhose *f*
- cirrhosis of the liver = cirrhose du foie
citric acid   acide *m* citrique
claustrophobia   claustrophobie *f*
clavicle; collarbone   clavicule *f*
cleansing lotion; cleansing milk   lait *m* de toilette; lait *m* démaquillant
clear (to) (eg throat, nose, chest)   dégager *v*
cleft palate   palais *m* fendu
clinic (private hospital)   clinique *f*
- maternity hospital/home = clinique d'accouchement
clinical   clinique *adj*
- clinical sign = signe *m* clinique
clip; agraffe   agrafe *f*
clitoris   clitoris *m*
clone   clone *m*
clone (to)   cloner *v*
clot; blood clot   caillot *m* sanguin
- a thrombosis = une thrombose
club-foot; talipes   pied-bot *m*
coagulant   coagulant *m*
coagulation   coagulation *f*
coagulation time   temps *m* de coagulation
cocaine   cocaïne *f*

coccyx coccyx *m*
cochlear cochléaire *adj*
cochlea {AM: spiral cavity of internal ear] **cochlée** *f* (syn. limaçon osseux) [AM: cavité
  enroulé en spirale de l'oreille interne]
cod liver oil huile *f* de foie de morue
codeine codéine *f*
coil; IUD; intra-uterine device stérilet *m*
cold rhume *m*; rhume simple; rhume de cerveau
cold in the head; coryza; rhinitis coryza *m*
cold sore bouton *m* de fièvre
cold sores; herpes simplex herpès *m* buccal
colibacillosis colibacillose *f*
colic, biliary; colic, hepatic colique *f* hépatique
colic, renal; colic, nephritic colique *f* néphrétique
colic; gripes; tormina; after-pains (of childbirth) tranchées *fpl*
colitis [AM: inflammation of the colon] colite *f* [AM: inflammation du colon]
collagen collagène *m*; also *adj*
collar (surgical) minerve *f*
collarbone; clavicule clavicule *f*
Colles' fracture Pouteau-Colles, fracture *f* de
colon côlon *m*
  ▪ irritable colon = côlon irritable
coloscopy [AM: visual examination of interior of colon] coloscopie *f* [AM: examen visuel
  de l'intérieur du côlon]
colour blindness; daltonism daltonisme *m*
colour-blind person; colour-blind daltonien *m*; daltonienne *f*; also *adj*
coma coma *m*
  ▪ brain-dead = dans un coma dépassé
  ▪ to be/ to go into a coma = être/entrer dans le coma
comb peigne *m*
  ▪ fine-tooth comb (for headlice) = peigne à poux
complete breech presentation siege *m* complet
complications complications *fpl*
compress compresse *f*
compress, antiseptic compresse *f* désinfectante
compress (to) compresser *v*
compression of the spinal column tassement *m* de la colonne (vertébrale)
compressive compressif,-ive *adj*
conception conception *f*
concretion (eg of a calculus) concrétion *f*
concussion commotion *f*

- concussion = commotion cérébrale
conditioner conditionneur *m*
condom préservatif *m*
confinement (eg to a mental hospital) internement *m*
confinement; childbirth couches *fpl*
  - a woman in labour = une femme en couches
  - miscarriage = fausse couche
  - resumption of menses (after childbirth) = retour de couches
  - she had a difficult labour = elle a eu des couches pénibles
  - to die in childbirth = mourir en couches
congenital congénital,-e *adj*
congenital ailments/diseases affections *fpl* congénitales
congestion congestion *f*
  - congestion of the lungs = congestion pulmonaire
  - stroke (cerebrovascular accident) = congestion cérébrale
conjunctiva [AM: membrane of the eyelid] conjonctive *f* [AM: membrane de la paupière]
conjunctivitis [AM: inflammation of the conjunctiva] conjonctivite *f* [AM: inflammation de la conjonctive]
consanguinity consanguinité *f*
consciousness connaisance *f*
  - he remained unconscious for an hour = il est resté sans connaisance pendant une heure
  - to become unconscious = perdre connaissance
  - to faint = tomber sans connaissance
constipate (to); make constipated (to) constiper *v*
  - constipated = constipé,-e (*adj*)
  - person suffering constipation = constipé *m*; constipée *f*
constipation constipation *f*
constitution constitution *f*
consultation consultation
  - outpatients' clinic = service (hospitalier) de consultation externe
  - to visit the surgery; to visit the doctor's office = aller à la consultation
consulting room cabinet *m* de consultation
contact contact *m*
  - it's contagious = ça s'attrape par le contact
contact lenses lentilles *fpl* de contact
contagion; cantagiousness contagion *f*
contaminate (to) contaminer *v*
  - contaminated = contaminé
contaminate (to) (blood) corrompre *v* (sang)
contraception contraception *f*

contraceptive contraceptif m; anticonceptionnel m; also adj
contraceptive pill pilule f anticonceptionnelle; pilule contraceptive
- I am on the pill = je prends la pilule
- I have come off the pill = j'ai arrêté la pilule

contraction contraction f
contraction (eg of pupil); shrinking; stricture (eg of heart); stenosis
rétrécissement m
- narrowing of the aortic valve = rétrécissement de la valve aortique

contracture [AM: involuntary prolonged muscular contraction, eg cramp]
contracture f [AM: contraction involontaire prolongée des muscles, par ex.
crampe]

contraindication contre-indication f
- the contraindications of a medicine = les contre-indications d'un medicament

convalescence convalescence f
convalescent home centre m de convalescence
convulsion convulsion f
cord cordon m
- medullary cords = cordons de la moelle épinière
- spermatic cord = cordon spermatique
- spinal cord = cordon médullaire
- umbilical cord = cordon ombilical

corn (on foot) cor m
- corn plaster (protector) = cor emplâtre
- corn plaster (remover/softener) = pansement pour le cor

cornea (eye) cornée f
coronary coronaire adj
coronary heart disease maladie f coronarienne
coronary thrombosis infarctus m du myocarde; thrombose f coronarienne
corpulence; stoutness corpulence f
- of slight/stout/medium build = de faible/forte/moyenne corpulence

correct (to) (eg vision) corriger v
cortex cortex m
- the cerebral cortex = le cortex cérébral

cortisone cortisone f
cotton wool coton m; ouate f
- cotton wool; absorbent cotton = ouate hydrophile
- make-up remover pad = coton démaquillant
- surgical cotton wool; surgical cotton = ouate chirurgicale

cotton-bud; cotton applicator coton-tige ® m
cough toux f
- dry cough = toux seche

- she has a bad cough = elle a une mauvaise toux
- smoker's cough = toux de fumeur

cough (to)   tousser *v*
- cough ! = toussez !

cough lozenge; cough tablet   pastille *f* pour la toux

cough mixture; cough syrup   antitussif *m*; sirop *m* antitussif; sirop *m* pour la toux

coughing   toux *f*

coughing fit   quinte *f* de toux

crack; chapping   gerçure *f*
- to have badly chapped hands = avoir les mains pleines de gerçures

cramp   crampe *f*
- I am having cramp(s) = j'ai des crampes
- I have a cramp in my leg = j'ai une crampe à la jambe
- stomach cramps = crampes d'estomac

cranium; skull   crâne *m*

cream   crème *f*
- anti-wrinkle cream= crème antirides
- antiseptic cream = crème antiseptique
- baby's cream = crème pour bébés
- cleansing cream = crème démaquillante
- cream for red skin/ erythema cream = crème antirougeurs
- day cream = crème de jour
- foundation cream = crème de base
- hair remover cream = crème dépilatoire; crème à épiler
- hand cream = crème pour les mains
- moisturising cream; moisturiser = crème hydratante
- nappy rash cream = crème contre les rougeurs
- shaving cream = crème à raser

crepitation; crackling   crépitation *f*
- articulary crepitation = crépitation articulaire
- bony crepitation; crepitus = crépitation osseuse
- crepitations = crépitation pulmonaire

cretinism   crétinisme *m*

Creutzfeldt-Jakob disease   Creutzfeldt-Jakob, maladie de

Crohn's disease   [AM: chronic enteritis affecting terminal part of ileum]   Crohn, maladie
de; iléite *f* régionale   [AM: inflammation chronique de l'iléon terminal]

croup   croup *m*

crown (of tooth)   couronne *f*
- dental crown; capping = couronne dentaire

crutch   béquille *f*
- forearm crutch = béquille d'avant-bras; canne anglaise

- underarm crutch = béquille commune

cupping glass; ventouse ventouse *f*

curable guérissable *adj*

curare curare *m*

cure guérison *f*

cure (to) (eg illness); make better (to); heal (to) (eg a wound) guérir *v*

curettage curetage *m*; curettage *m*

curette; scraper curette *f*

curvature of the spine déviation *f* de la colonne vertébrale

Cushing's syndrome [AM: syndrome due to the overproduction of glucocorticoids]
syndrome de Cushing [AM: syndrome causé par l'hyperproduction de glucocorticoïdes]

Cushing's disease maladie *f* de Cushing

cut coupure *f*

cyanosis cyanose *f*

cycling cyclisme *m*

- to do a lot of cycling = faire beaucoup de vélo

cyst kyste *m*; loupe *f*

cystic kystique *adj*

cystic fibrosis fibrose *f* kystique

cystitis [AM: inflammation of the bladder] cystite *f* [AM: inflammation de la vessie]

cytobacteriological examination (eg of urine) examen *m* cytobactério-logique

D

damage (to) (eg hands) abîmer *v*

- hépatite peut abîmer le foie = hepatitis can damage the liver

damage (to); injure (to) léser *v*

dance danse *f*

- to have St Vitus's dance = avoir la danse de Saint-Guy

dandruff pellicules *fpl*

- dandruff lotion = lotion contre les pellicules

dazzle éblouissement *m*

- to have a dizzy turn/spell = avoir un éblouissement/étourdissement

dead person mort *f*

deaf sourd,-e *adj*

deaf-aid appareil *m* acoustique; audiophone *m*

deafness surdité *f*

death mort *f*; décès *m*

- brain death = mort cérébrale/mort clinique/mort relative
- clinical death = mort absolue/mort définitive
- natural death = mort naturelle
- sudden infant death = mort subite imprévue du nourrisson

decibel (dB) [AM: unit of sound intensity] décibel *m* (dB) [AM: unité de mesure de l'intensité sonore]

decompression sickness maladie *f* des caissons

decongest (to); relieve congestion in (to) décongestionner *v*

decongestant décongestionnant *m*; décongestif *m*; décongestif,-ve *adj*

defecation défécation *f*

defibrillate (to) défibriller *v*

defibrillation défibrillation *f*

defibrillator défibrillateur *m*

deficiency carence *f*
- deficiency disease = maladie de/par carence
- vitamin deficiency = carence vitaminique; carence en vitamines

deficiency déficience *f*
- immunodeficiency = déficience immunologique
- mental deficiency = déficience mentale
- muscular insufficiency = déficience musculaire

deficient person; deficient *(adj)* déficient *m*; déficient,-e *adj*
- mentally deficient child; child with physical disability = enfant déficient
- mentally/visually handicapped person = déficient mental/visuel

deformation déformation *f*

deformity difformité *f*; monstruosité *f*
- congenital deformity = difformité congénitale
- to be deformed = présenter des difformités

degenerating; deteriorating dégénérescent,-e *adj*

degeneration; deterioration dégénération *f*; dégénérescence *f*

degree degré *m*
- degree centigrade /Fahrenheit /Baumé = degré centigrade/Fahrenheit /Baumé
- degree of burns = degré de brûlure
- first/second degree burn = brûlure du premier/deuxième degré

dehydrated déshydraté,-e *adj*

dehydration déshydratation *f*

delirious (to be) délirer *v*

delirium délire *m*
- hallucinatory delirium = délire hallucinatoire
- persecution mania = délire de persécution

delirium tremens delirium tremens

deliver (a child) (to); give birth (to) accoucher *v*

descent

delivery; expulsion; freeing (of baby in childbirth) dégagement *m*
demented person; demented (*adj*) dément *m*; démente *f*; also *adj*
dementia; madness démence *f*
 ▪ dementia praecox = démence précoce
demulcent; emollient émollient *m*; émollient,-e *adj*
demulcent; softener adoucissant *m*; adoucissant,-e *adj*
dengue (fever); breakbone fever dengue *f*
dental dentaire *adj*; dental -e *adj*
dental amalgam amalgame *m* dentaire
dental floss fil *m* dentaire
dental plaque plaque *f* dentaire
dental plate dentier *m*
dental pulp pulpe *f* dentaire
dental technician; dental mechanic mécanicien-dentiste *m*
dental treatment traitement *m* dentaire
dentine dentine *f*
dentist dentiste *m/f*
 ▪ a dental appointment = un rendez-vous chez le dentiste
 ▪ I need to see a dentist = j'ai besoin de voir un dentiste
 ▪ to go to the dentist = s'aller chez le dentiste
dentistry dentisterie *f*; odontologie *f*
dentition denture *f*; dentier *m*
denture prothèse *f* dentaire; dentier *m*
 ▪ my dentures are broken = mon dentier est cassé
 ▪ can you repair them? = vous pouvez le réparer?
deodorant; antiperspirant déodorant *m*
 ▪ spray-on deodorant = déodorant en spray
 ▪ stick deodorant = déodorant en stick
depilatory dépilatoire *m*
deposit dépôt *m*
depressed person; neurasthenic neurasthénique *m,f*
depression dépression *f*
 ▪ nervous breakdown = dépression nerveuse
 ▪ neurotic depression = dépression névrotique
 ▪ post-operative depression = dépression opératoire
 ▪ slight/moderate depression = dépression légère/modérée
dermatitis [AM: skin affection] dermatite *f*, dermite *f* [AM: affection cutanée]
dermatological bulla; large skin blister bulle *f* dermatologique
dermatologiste dermatologiste *m,f*
dermatology dermatologie *f*
descent descente *f*

- prolapse of an organ = descente d'organe
desensitization désensibilisation *f*
desensitize (to) désensibiliser *v*
detachment (eg of retina) décollement *m*
- detachment of the retina = décollement de la rétine
detangling; untangling (hair) démêlant,-e *adj*
- detangling preparation/balm = baume démêlant
detect (to) (eg a disease) dépister *v*
detoxification désintoxication *f*
detoxify (to) désintoxiquer *v*
development; evolution évolution *f*
deviation; inversion (of an organ); displacement (of uterus); curvature (of spine) déviation *f*
dextrose dextrose *m*
diabetes diabète *m*
- diabetes insipidus = diabète insipide
- diabetes mellitus = diabète sucré
- latent diabetes = diabète latent
- to have diabetes; to suffer from diabetes = faire diabète
- to have diabetes = être diabétique
diabetic diabétique *adj*
- I am diabetic = je suis diabétique
diagnose (to) diagnostiquer *v*
diagnosis diagnostic *m*; diagnose *f*
diagnostic diagnostique *adj*
diagnostic computer ordinateur *m* de diagnostic
dialyser dialyseur *m*
dialysis épuration *f* extrarénale
dialysis machine rein *m* artificiel (syn. hémodialyseur *m*)
dialysis unit unité *f* de dialyse
diaphragm diaphragme *m*
diarrhoea colique *f*
- I have diarrhoea; stomach pain; colic pain; colic = j'ai les coliques
diarrhoea diarrhée *f*
- acute attack of diarrhoea = turista *f*
- I've got diarrhoea = j'ai la diarrhée
- travellers' diarrhoea = diarrhée des voyageurs
diet diète *f*
diet; system; regime régime *m*
- health insurance scheme = régime maladie
- hospital system/regulations = régime des hôpitaux

- slimming diet = régime amaigrissant
- Social Security system = régime de la Sécurité sociale
- to be on a diet = suivre un régime

dietician diététicien *m*; diététicienne *f*
dietist diétiste *m*
digest (to) digérer *v*
digestibility digestibilité *f*
digestible digestible *adj*
digestion digestion *f*
digestive digestif,-ive *adj*
digestive glands glandes *fpl* digestives
digestive system système *m* digestif; appareil *m* digestif
digitalis digitaline *f*
dilation; dilatation dilatation *f*
- dilation of the pupil = dilatation de la pupille

dilator; dilatator dilatateur *m*; also *adj*
diphtheria diphtérie *f*
diplegia diplégie *f*
disability; handicap handicap *m*
disabled person handicapé *m*; handicapée *f*
disabled person; disabled (adj) invalide *m,f* also *adj*
disc disque *m*
- intervertebral disc = disque intervertébral

disc, of an invertebratal discal,-e *adj*
- slipped disc = hernie discale

discharge (of patient) décharge *f*; démission *f*; licenciement *m*
disease; affection maladie *f*; affection *f*
disinfect (to) désinfecter *v*
disinfectant désinfectant *m*; désinfectant,-e *adj*
- disinfectant = produit *m* désinfectant

disinfecting ointment; germicidal ointment pommade *f* anti-infection
disinfection désinfection *f*
dislocate (to) se disloquer *v*; se luxer *v*; se déboîter *v*
- dislocated = disloqué,-e *adj*
- to dislocate one's knee = se déboîter le genou
- to dislocate one's shoulder = se disloquer l'épaule

dislocation dislocation *f*; luxation *f*; déboîtement *m*
disorder désordre *m*
- functional/liver disorder = désordre fonctionnel/hépatique

disorientation désorientation *f*
displace (to) (eg a joint) déplacer *v*

- to put a joint out; to displace a joint = se déplacer une articulation
- to slip a disc = se déplacer une vertèbre

distension (eg stomach) gonflement *m*

district nurse; visiting nurse infirmière *f* visiteuse; infirmière visitante

diuretic diurétique *m*; also *adj*

diverticulitis [AM: inflammation of diverticula of the colon] diverticulite *f* [AM: inflammation des diverticules du côlon]

diverticulum diverticule *m*

dizziness; vertigo; giddiness vertige *m*
- I feel dizzy = j'ai des vertiges
- to suffer from vertigo = avoir des vertiges

doctor docteur *m*
- doctor of medicine = docteur en médecine

doctor; physician médecin *m*
- army medical officer = médecin militaire
- company doctor = médecin du travail
- consultant = médecin d'hôpital
- family practitioner/doctor = médecin de famille
- forensic scientist = médecin légiste
- general practitioner (G.P.) = médecin généraliste
- medical adviser = médecin-conseil
- school doctor = médecin scolaire

doctor's fee honoraires *mpl* de médecin

dome of the skull; calvaria voûte *f* crânienne; calotte *f* crânienne

donation of organs don *m* d'organes

donor donneur *m*; donneuse *f*
- blood donor = donneur de sang

dopamine dopamine *f*

dorsal dorsal,-e *adj.*

dorsal vertebra vertèbre *f* dorsale

dosage posologie *f*

dose (eg of medicine) dose *f*

dose up (to); give drugs to (to) droguer *v*
- to take drugs; to be on drugs = se droguer

douche douche *f* vaginale; lavage *m* interne

Down's syndrome; mongolism syndrome de Down; mongolisme *m*

Down's syndrome; with Down's syndrome mongolien,-ienne *adj*

drain (to) drainer *v*

drain; drainage tube drain *m*

drainage drainage *m*
- lymphatic drainage = drainage lymphatique

dream rêve *m*

dress (to) (a wound); put a dressing on (to); bandage (to) panser *v*; mettre un pansement/un bandage à/sur

dressing, sterilized compresse *f* stérilisée

dressing; bandage pansement *m*
- compressive bandage = pansement compressif
- dry/moist dressing = pansement sec/humide

drip feeding drip *m* feeding

drip transfusion drip *m* transfusion

drip; IV (US); perfusion perfusion *f*
- to put someone on a drip or an IV (US) = mettre quelqu'un sous perfusion

drop (of liquid) goutte *f*
- drip = goutte-à-goutte *m inv*
- to be drip-fed = être nourri au goutte-à-goutte
- to have a dripping or runny nose = avoir la goutte au nez

dropper compte-gouttes *m*

dropsy [AM: general oedema of the tissues] hydropisie *f* (terme mod. 'anasarque') [AM: œdème généralisé du tissu]

drowning noyade *f*
- death by drowning = mort *f* par noyade

drowsiness; somnolence somnolence *f*

drug; narcotic drogue *f*; narcotique *m*; also *adj*; stupéfiant *m*; stupéfiant,-e *adj*
- hard/soft drug = drogue dure/ douce

drug addict drogué *m*; droguée *f*; intoxiqué *m*; intoxiquée *f*; toxicomane *m,f*

drug addiction toxicomanie *f*

drug; narcotic narcotique *m*; also *adj*; stupéfiant *m*; stupéfiant,-e *adj*

duct; pathway; tract voie *f*

dumbness; muteness; mutism mutisme *m*; mutité *f*

dummy; pacifier; comforter sucette *f*; tétine *f*

duodenitis [AM: inflammation of the duodenum] duodénite *f* [AM: inflammation du duodénum]

duodenum [AM: part of the intestine] duodénum *m* [AM: partie de l'intestin]

duration of hospitalisation durée *f* de l'hospitalisation

dwarfism; nanism nanisme *m*

dye, hair teinture *f* pour les cheveux
- to dye one's hair = se teindre les cheveux

dysentery dysenterie *f*

dysfunction dysfonction *f*; dysfonctionnement *m*

dyslexia dyslexie *f*

dyslexic person dyslexique *m,f*; also *adj*

dysmenorrhoea dysménorrhée *f*

dyspepsia dyspepsie *f*

138

dysphasia dysphasie *f*
dystrophy [AM: defective nutrition leading to wasting of tissue] dystrophie *f* [AM: nutrition
  déficiente entraînant dégénérescence du tissu]
  ▪ muscular dystrophy = dystrophie musculaire
dysuria [AM: difficulty in urinating] dysurie *f* [AM: difficulté à uriner]

E

ear oreille *f*
  ▪ external ear; auricle = oreille externe
  ▪ internal ear = oreille interne
ear drops gouttes *fpl* pour les oreilles
ear infection; otitis; earache otite *f*
ear lobe lobe *m* de l'oreille
ear plugs protège-tympan *m*
  ▪ ear plug (for noise) = boule Quiès ® (pour bruit)
  ▪ ear plug (for water) = bouchon d'oreille (pour l'eau)
ear, nose and throat department département *m* d'oto-rhino-laryngologie;
  service *m* d'oto-rhino-laryngologie
ear, nose and throat specialist oto-rhino-laryngologiste *m,f*
earache mal *m* aux oreilles; mal d'oreilles
eardrum tympan *m*
ease (to); relieve (to) calmer *v*; soulager *v*
eau de Cologne eau *f* de Cologne
eau de parfum eau *f* de parfum
eau de toilette eau *f* de toilette
Ebola virus disease maladie *f* à virus Ebola
echocardiography; ultrasound cardiography échocardiographie *m*
eclampsia éclampsie *f*
eczema eczéma *m*
effect effet *m*
  ▪ side effects = effets secondaires
effectiveness; efficacy efficacité *f*
  ▪ therapeutic effectiveness = efficacité thérapeutique
effleurage; light massage effleurage *m*
  ▪ to touch/massage lightly = effleurer
effusion épanchement *m*
  ▪ to have water on the knee = avoir un épanchement de synovie

139

elastic support bandage   bande *f* de tissu élastique
elbow   coude *m*
elderly   les personnes *fpl* âgées
electric shock (see also shock)   décharge *f* électrique
electrocardiogram   électrocardiogramme *m*
electrocardiograph   électrocardiographe *m*
electrocardiography   électrocardiographie *f*, ECG
electroencephalogram; EEG   [AM: graphical trace of electrical activity of the brain]
   électroencéphalogramme *m*; EEG   [AM: trace graphique des rythmes électriques cérébraux]
electroencephalograph   électroencéphalographe *m*
electroencephalography   électroencéphalographie *f*, EEG
electronic monitoring   surveillance *f* électronique
electronic thermometer   thermomètre *m* électronique
electrotherapy   électrothérapie *f*
eliminate (to)   éliminer *v*
elimination   élimination *f*
embolism   embolie *f*
 ▪ arterial embolism = embolie artérielle
 ▪ cerebral embolism = embolie cérébrale
embrocation   embrocation *f*
embryo   embryon *m*
 ▪ frozen embryo = embryon congelé
embryology   embryologie *f*
embryonic   embryonnaire *adj*
emergency   urgence *f*
 ▪ medical emergency = une urgence médicale
 ▪ the casualty department; casualty = le service des urgences
 ▪ the casualty department; casualty = les urgences
emetic   émétique *m*
emotion   émotion *f*
emphysema   emphysème *m*
 ▪ emphysema of the lungs = emphysème pulmonaire
empiric; empirical   empirique *m*; empirique *adj*
 ▪ empirical remedy = remède empirique
emulsion   émulsion *f*
enamel (tooth)   émail *m*
encephalitis   [AM: inflammation of the brain]   encéphalite *f*   [AM: inflammation de l'encéphale]
encephalogram   encéphalogramme *m*
encephalon   encéphale *m*

endemic endémique *adj*

endocarditis [AM: inflammation of the endocardium]   endocardite *f* [AM: inflammation de l'endocarde]

endocardium (of heart) endocarde *m*

endocrine gland glande *f* endocrine

endocrine system; endocrine glands système *m* endocrinien

endocrinology endocrinologie *f*

endogenous [AM: produced from within (the body)]   endogène *adj* [AM: qui est dû à des causes interne]

endometritis [AM: inflammation of the uterine lining]   endométrite *f* [AM: inflammation de la muqueuse utérine]

endometrium [AM: lining membrane of uterus]   endomètre *m* [AM: muqueuse tapissant la face interne de l'utérus]

endoscope [AM: instrument for inspecting interior of a cavity]   endoscope *m* [AM: instrument permettant d'observer l'intérieur d'une cavité]

endoscopy endoscopie *f*

enema; rectal injection lavement *m*
  ▪ barium enema (for radiological examination) = lavement baryté

engorge (to); obstruct (to) engorger *v*

engorgement; obstruction engorgement *m*

enteritis [AM: inflammation of the lining of the small intestine]   entérite *f* [AM: inflammation de la muqueuse de l'intestin grêle]

enterobacteria entérobactérie *f*

enterobiasis; oxyuriasis oxyurose *f*

enterocolitis entérocolite *f*

enterovirus entérovirus *m*

enzyme enzyme *f* ou *m*

epicondylitis; tennis elbow épicondylite *f*

epidemic épidémie *f*

epidermis épiderme *m*

epididymis épididyme *m*

epiglottis épiglotte *f*

epilepsy épilepsie *f*

epileptic épileptique *m,f*

epileptic épileptique *adj*
  ▪ epileptic fit = crise *f* d'épilepsie

epistaxis [AM: nose bleeding]   épistaxis *f* [AM: saignement de nez]

epithelial épithélial,-e *adj*
  ▪ epithelial tissue = tissu épithélial

epithelioma; carcinoma [AM: malignant tumour of epithelial tissue]   épithélioma *m*; épithéliome *m* [AM: tumeur maligne d'un tissu épithélial]

epithelium [AM: membranous tissue covering most internal/external surfaces] épithélium *m*

eye socket

[AM: tissu de revêtement qui recouvre les surfaces internes/externes]
erratic erratique *adj*
eruption (of a tooth) éruption *f*
erysipelas [AM: streptoccocal infection of the skin]   érysipèle *m*; érésipèle *m*
   [AM: maladie streptococcique de la peau]
erythema érythème *m*
erythremia maladie de Vaquez
erythrocyte [AM: red blood cell]   érythrocyte *m*; globule *m* rouge; hématie [AM: cellule
   sanguine rouge]
erythromycin [AM: antibiotic]   érythromycine *f* [AM: antibiotique]
euthanasia euthanasie *f*
evacuate (to); discharge (to) évacuer *v*
evacuation évacuation *f*
evacuation; defecation déjection *f*
   ▪ faeces; excrement = déjections
eventration; rupture éventration *f*
evolve (to); develop (to) évoluer *v*
   ▪ the illness is running its (normal) course = la maladie évolue
examination examen *m*
   ▪ clinical examination = examen clinique
   ▪ complementary examination (eg. blood analysis, radiography) = examen
      complémentaire
   ▪ medical examination = examen médical
   ▪ pre-marital examination = examen prénuptial
   ▪ sight test = examen de la vue
examination room local *m* d'examens; salle *f* d'examens
examine (to) examiner *v*
excite (to); stimulate (to) (eg nerve, muscle) exciter *v*
excressence; outgrowth excroissance *f*
excretion excrétion *f*
exercise bicycle vélo *m* d'entrainement; vélo d'appartement
exhaustion épuisement *m;* coup *m* de pompe
exit; discharge (of patient) sortie *f*
expectorant expectorant *m*; also *adj*
external; exterior externe *adj*
external bleeding hémorragie *f* externe
extract (to); pull out (to) (eg tooth) arracher *v*; extraire *v*
   ▪ I don't want it (tooth) extracted = je ne voudrais pas me le faire arracher
extraction extraction *f*
eye œil *m*; yeux *mpl*
eye shadow ombre *m* à paupières
eye socket; orbit orbite *f*

142

eye specialist oculiste *m,f*; ophtalmologiste *m,f*; ophtalmologue *m*
eye surgery chirurgie *f* ophtalmique
eye unit; ophthalmology unit unité *f* ophtalmologique
eye wash; eye lotion collyre *m*
eyeball globe *m* oculaire
eyebath; eyecup œillère *f*
eyebrow sourcil *m*
eyebrow pencil crayon *m* à sourcils
eyedrops gouttes *fpl* pour les yeux
eyelash cil *m*
eyelid paupière *f*
 ■ lower/upper eyelid = paupière inférieure/supérieure
eyeliner crayon *m* pour les yeux
eyes yeux *mpl*
eyesight; vision vision *f*; vue *f*

F

face face *f*; visage *m*
face pack masque *m* de beauté
 ■ mud pack = masque *m* de beauté à l'argile
facial soins *mpl* du visage
 ■ I would like a facial = je voudrai des soins du visage
factor facteur *m*
 ■ Rhesus or Rh factor = facteur Rhésus
faint (to) évanouir *v*; s'évanouir
 ■ unconscious = évanoui *adj*
fainting fit; fainting spell; blackout évanouissement *m*
Fallopian tube trompe *f* de Fallope
false teeth fausses dents *fpl*
family planning planification *f* familiale; planning *m* familial
fantasy; delusion fantasme *m*
fast (to) jeûner *v*
fasting; abstention from food jeûne *m*
fatigue fatigue *f*
 ■ chronic fatigue syndrome = syndrome de fatigue chronique
fatty acids acides *mpl* gras
 ■ monounsaturated fatty acids = les acides gras monoinsaturés

- polyunsaturated fatty acids = les acides gras polyinsaturés
- saturated fatty acids = les acides gras saturés
- unsaturated fatty acids = les acides gras insaturés

features; facies faciès *m*

febrifuge fébrifuge *m; also adj*; antipyrétique *m; also adj*

feel (to) sentir *v*
- I don't feel well = je ne me sens pas bien

feeling of sickness or fainting malaise *m*
- to feel faint ou dizzy = avoir un malaise

femoral (eg artery, nerve) fémoral *adj*

femur [AM: thigh bone] fémur *m* [AM: os de la cuisse]

fertility fécondité *f;* fertilité *f*

fertility drug médicament *m* contre la stérilité

fertilization fécondation *f*
- in vitro fertilization = fécondation in vitro

fever fièvre *f*
- he has a high temperature = il a beaucoup de fièvre
- I have a fever/ a high temperature = j'ai de la fièvre
- my temperature is 38 degrees = j'ai 38 de fièvre

feverish fiévreux, fiévreuse *adj*
- I feel feverish = je me sens fiévreux (homme)/ fiévreuse (femme)

fibrillation fibrillation *f*
- auricular fibrillation = fibrillation auriculaire
- ventricular fibrillation = fibrillation ventriculaire

fibrositis fibrosite *f,* aponévrite *f*

fibula (leg bone) péroné *m*

field of vision; visual field champ *m* visuel; champ *m* de vision

filling (tooth) plombage *m*
- a filling has fallen out = un plombage a sauté
- I have lost a filling = j'ai perdu un plombage
- the filling has come out = le plombage est parti

finger doigt *m*
- little finger = petit doigt
- mallet finger = doigt en marteau

fingernail ongle *m*; ongle *m* de la main
- brittle nails = ongles cassants
- well-manicured nails = ongles soignés

fingerstall doightier *m*

first aid premiers soins *mpl*; prompts secours *mpl*

first aid box/kit trousse *f* d'urgence; trousse *f* à/de premier secours

first aid manual manuel *m* de premiers soins

fist poing *m*

fistula   fistule *f*
flannel; face-flannel   gant *m* de toilette
flat   plat,-e *adj*
- to have flat feet = avoir les pieds plats
flatulence   flatulence *f*
flatus   flatuosité *f*
- to have wind = avoir des flatuosités
flavour   parfum *m*
flex (to)   fléchir *v*
flourine   fluor *m*
flow   flux *m*
- flow of blood = flux de sang
- menstrual flow = flux menstruel
flu; influenza   grippe *f*; affection *f* grippale; état *m* grippal
fluke   distome *m*; douve *f*
fluoridation   fluoration *f*
fluoride   fluorure *m*
fluoroscopy   radioscopie *f*
flush   flush *m*
foetus   fœtus *m*
folic acid   acide *m* folique
follicle   follicule *m*
folliculitis   folliculite *f*
fontanelle   [AM: non-bony part of baby's head]   fontanelle *f* [AM: espace membraneux, non ossifié du crâne de nouveau-né]
food poisoning   intoxication *f* alimentaire
food supplement   complément *m* alimentaire
foot   pied *m*
- athlete's foot = mycose du pied
- club-foot = pied bot
- flat foot; pes valgus = pied plat
- hollow foot; pes cavus = pied creux
forceps; pair of forceps   forceps *m*; fers *mpl*
forearm   avant-bras *m*
forearm crutch   béquille *f* d'avant-bras
forehead   front *m*
forensic medicine   médecine *f* légale
formication; pins and needles   fourmillement *m*
foundation (cosmet)   fond *m* de teint
fracture   fracture *f*
- compound fracture; open fracture = fracture ouverte
- compound fracture = fracture compliquée

- fractured skull; fracture of the skull = fracture du crâne
- simple fracture; closed fracture = fracture fermée

fracture (to)   fracturer *v*
- he fractured his leg = il s'est fracturé la jambe

frank breech presentation   siege *m* décomplété

free radical   radical *m* libre

friction massage, localised   frictions *fpl* localisées

front teeth   dents *fpl* de devant

frostbite   gelure *f*

fumigator   fumigateur *m*

fungus; mushroom   champignon *m*
- hallucinogenic mushroom; magic mushroom = champignon hallucinogène
- poisonous toadstool = champignon vénéneux

furuncle   clou *m*; furoncle *m*

G

gall bladder   vésicule *f* biliaire

gall stone; bile stone   calcul *m* biliaire

gamma rays   rayons *mpl* gamma

ganglion   ganglion *m*
- lymph gland = ganglion lymphatique
- to have swollen glands = avoir des ganglions

gangrene   gangrène *f*

gargle (to)   gargariser *v*; se gargariser *v*

gargle; mouthwash   gargarisme *m*
- to gargle = se faire un gargarisme

gargling   gargarisme *m*

gastrectomy   [AM: removal of part or whole of the stomach]   gastrectomie *f*   [AM: résection partielle ou totale de l'estomac]

gastric   gastrique *adj*

gastric acidity   acidité *f* gastrique

gastric flu   grippe *f* gastro-intestinale

gastric ulcer   ulcère *m* de l'estomac

gastritis   [AM: inflammation of the stomach lining]   gastrite *f*   [AM: inflammation de la muqueuse de l'estomac]

gastro-enterology department   service *m* de gastro-entérologie

gastroenteritis   [AM: inflammation of lining of stomach and the intestine]   gastroentérite *f*

[AM: inflammation des muqueuses de l'estomac et de l'intestin]

gauze   gaze *f*
- cotton gauze = gaze de coton

gel, shower   gel *m* douche

gelatin capsule   gélule *f*

gene   gène *m*

gene therapy   thérapie *f* genique

general practitioner; family doctor   médecin *m* de famille; médecin *m* généraliste

generalize (to)   généraliser *v*
- general cancer = cancer généralisé
- systemic infection = infection généralisée
- to spread (eg disease) = se généraliser

genetic code   code *m* génétique

genetic engineering   génie *m* génétique

genetics; genetic (adj)   génétique *f*, also *adj*

genitalia; genital organs   organes *mpl* génitaux

genome   génome *m*
- human genome = génome humain

geriatric   gériatrique *adj*

geriatric department   service *m* gériatrique

geriatrics   gériatrie *f*

germ   germe *m*

gerontology   gérontologie *f*

gestation; pregnancy   gestation *f*

giddiness   étourdissement *m*

gingivitis   [AM: inflammation of the gums]   gingivite *f* [AM: inflammation des gencives]

ginkgo biloba   ginkgo biloba *m*
- ginkgo extract = ginkgolide *m*

ginseng   ginseng *m*

give (someone) a shock (to)   commotionner *v* (quelqu'un)
- he has received a severe electric shock = une décharge électrique l'a commotionné
- in a state of shock; suffering from concussion = commotionné
- to be severely shocked = être fortement commotionné

give birth to (a baby) (to)   accoucher de *v*

gland   glande *f*

glanders   morve *f*

glandular   glandulaire *adj*

glandular fever   mononucléose *f* infectieuse

glasses   lunettes *fpl*
- bifocal glasses = lunettes bifocales

147

- dark glasses = lunettes noires
- sunglasses = lunettes de soleil

Glauber's salt (sodium sulfate) sel *m* de Glauber

glaucoma glaucome *m*

glottis glotte *f*

gloves, latex gants *mpl* latex

glucose glucose *m*

glucose tolerance test épreuve *f* de tolérance au glucose; épreuve d' hyper-glycémie f provoquée

gluten gluten *m*

glycerine glycérine *f* (syn. glycérol *m*)

goitre; goiter goitre *m*

gonad gonade *f*

gonorrhea; gonococcal urethritis gonorrhée *f*; blennorragie *f*; échauffement *m*

gout goutte *f*

grain; pellet grain *m*

gravel; urinary calculus gravelle *f*; lithiase *f* urinaire

graze; scratch éraflure *f*

- to graze/scratch oneself = s'erafler

gripe water calmant *m* pour coliques infantiles

gripe; gripes coliques *fpl*

groin aine *f*

group therapy thérapie *f* de groupe

growth (eg of a child) croissance *f*

gum (of teeth) gencive *f*

- gums = les gencives

gum; gumma (pathological) gomme *f*

gustative; gustatory gustatif,-ive *adj*

gymnasium gymnase *m*

gymnast gymnaste *m,f*

gymnastics gymnastique *f*

- aquagym = gymnastique aquatique
- callisthenics = gymnastique suédoise
- eurythmics = gymnastique rhythmique et sportive; GRS
- physiotherapy exercises = gymnastique corrective

gynaecologist gynécologiste *m,f*; gynécologue *m,f*

gynaecology; gynecology gynécologie *f*

gynaecology unit unité *f* gynécologique

H

haematological hématologique *adj*
haematologist hématologiste *m,f*; hématologue *m,f*
haematology; hematology hématologie *f*
haematoma hématoma *m*
haemodialysis; hemodialysis hémodialyse *f*
haemoglobin; hemoglobin hémoglobine *f*
haemolysis hémolyse *f*
haemophilia hémophilie *f*
haemophiliac hémophile *m,f*
haemophilic hémophile *adj*
haemorrhage; bleeding hémorragie *f*
haemorrhagic hémorragique *adj*
haemorrhoidal; with haemorrhoids hémorroïdal,-e *adj*; hémorroïdaire *adj*
haemorrhoids; hemorrhoids hémorroïdes *fpl*
- I have haemorrhoids = j'ai des hémorroïdes
hair (body) poil *m*
hair (head) cheveux *mpl*
- loss of hair = chute des cheveux
hair clippers; hair trimmer tondeuse *f* à cheveux
hair conditioner après-shampooing *m*
hair curler bigoudi *m*
hair dye teinture *f* pour les cheveux
hair gel gel *m* coiffant
hair grip pince *f* à cheveux
hair loss, to cause; remove hair from (to) dépiler *v*
hair lotion lotion *f* capillaire
hair mousse mousse *f* coiffante; mousse *f* pour cheveux
hair net filet *m* à cheveux; résille *f*
hair remover; hair-removing; depilatory dépilatoire *m*; also *adj*
hair spray laque *f*; bombe *f* de laque
hairbrush brosse *f* à cheveux
hairclip; hair grip barrette *f*; pince *f* à cheveux
hairdryer sèche-cheveux *m*
hairpin épingle *f* à cheveux
halitosis; bad breath halitose *f*; mauvaise haleine *f*
hallucinated person halluciné *m*; hallucinée *f*
hallucination hallucination *f*
hallucinogenic hallucinogène *adj*
hand main *f*

- right/left hand = main droite/gauche
handicapped; disabled handicapé,-e *adj*
hangover gueule *f* de bois
harelip bec-de-lièvre *m*
hay fever rhume *m* des foins
head tête *f*
headache mal *m* à la tête; mal de tête; céphalée *f*; céphalalgie *f*
- tension headache = céphalée de tension
heal (to) cicatriser *v*
- ça devrait cicatriser rapidement = it should heal quickly
healing cicatrisant,-e *adj*
- healing product = cicatrisant *m*
healing cicatrisation *f*; guérison *f*
health santé *f*
health care protection *f* contre les maladies
health care centre centre *m* sanitaire
health care for mothers and young children protection *f* maternelle et infantile
health care service services *mpl* médicaux
health check-up bilan *m* de santé
health insurance; sickness benefit assurance *m* maladie
health record carnet *m* de santé
health; sanitary sanitaire *adj*
hearing; audition audition *f*; ouïe *f*
hearing aid prothèse *f* auditive; prothèse *f* acoustique; appareil *m* acoustique; audiophone *m*; audiphone *m*
heart cœur *m*
- I have a heart condition = j'ai le cœur malade
heart attack; coronary thrombosis; myocardial infarction infarctus *m* du myocarde
- to have a coronary; to have a heart attack = avoir un infarctus
heart disease maladie *f* du cœur
heart examination examen *m* cardiaque
heart rate (see also pulsation) fréquence *f* cardiaque; rythme *m* cardiaque
heart rate monitor moniteur *m* cardiaque
heart surgeon chirurgien *m* cardiaque; chirurgienne *f* cardiaque; cardio-chirurgien(ne)
heart surgery chirurgie *f* cardiaque
heartbeat rate; pulse rate fréquence *f* cardiaque
heartburn aigreurs *fpl* d'estomac; brûlures *fpl* d'estomac
heat exhaustion épuisement *m* dû à la chaleur
heatstroke coup *m* de chaleur

heel   talon *m*
height gauge   toise *f*
hemiplegia   [AM: paralysis of one side of the body]   hémiplégie *f* [AM: paralysie affectant une moitié du corps]
hemiplegic ; paralyzed on one side   hémiplégique *adj*
hemiplegic ; person paralyzed on one side   hémiplégique *m,f*
heparin   héparine *f*
hepatic   hépatique *adj*
hepatitis   hépatite *f*
- hepatitis A = hépatite A
- hepatitis B = hépatite B
- hepatitis C = hépatite C
- viral hepatitis = hépatite virale

herb, medicinal   herbe *f* médicinale
herbal medicine   médecine *f* par les plantes; phytothérapie *f*
hereditary disease   maladie *f* héréditaire
heredity   hérédité *f*
hernia; rupture   hernie *f*
- inguinal hernia = hernie inguinale
- slipped disc = hernie discale
- strangulated hernia = hernie étranglée

herpes   herpès *m*
- cold sore; herpes labialis = herpès de la lèvre
- genital herpes = herpès génital
- ringworm = herpès circiné

heterosexual   hétérosexuel *m*; hétérosexuelle *f*; also *adj*
heterosexuality   hétérosexualité *f*
hiccup (to); hiccough (to)   hoqueter *v*
hiccup; hiccough   hoquet *m*
- to have hiccups = avoir le hoquet

hinder (to); embarrass (to)   embarrasser *v*
- my tongue is coated = j'ai la langue embarrassée
- to have an upset stomach = avoir l'estomac embarrassé
- to lie heavy on the stomach = embarrasser l'estomac

hip   hanche *f*
hip bone   os *m* iliaque
hip joint; coxa   articulation *f* coxo-fémorale; articulation de la hanche
hip replacement   prothèse *f* de la hanche
hip replacement operation   pose *f* d'une prothèse de la hanche
hirsutism   hirsutisme *m*
histamine   histamine *f*

histology histologie *f*
hives; urticaria urticaire *f*
HIV-negative séronégativité *f*; séronégatif,-ive *adj*
HIV-positive séropositivité *f*; séropositif,-ive *adj*
Hodgkin's disease [AM: cancerous condition] Hodgkin, maladie *f* de [AM: affection cancéreuse]
holistic holistique *adj*
homeopathic homéopathique *adj*
  ▪ in small doses = à doses homéopathiques
homeopathy [AM: therapeutic method] homéopathie *f* [AM: méthode thérapeutique]
homosexual homosexuel *m*; homosexuelle *f*, also *adj*
homosexuality homosexualité *f*
hookworm ankylostome *m*
hookworm disease; ankylostomiasis; uncinariasis ankylostomiase *f*, ankylostomose *f*
hormone hormone *f*
hospital hôpital *m*
  ▪ children's hospital = hôpital *m* d'enfants
  ▪ general hospital = hôpital général
  ▪ out-patient clinic = hôpital de jour
  ▪ where is the hospital? = où est l'hôpital?
  ▪ you must go to hospital = il faut aller à l'hôpital
hospital training; period as houseman or intern; entrance examination (for hospital work) internat *m*
  ▪ during his/her period as an intern = pendant son internat
hospital trolley civière *f*
hot flush bouffée *f* de chaleur
hot-water bottle bouillotte *f*
house doctor; houseman interne *m,f* (des hôpitaux)
human body organisme *m*
  ▪ the body's natural defences = les défenses naturelles de l'organisme
human immunodeficiency virus; HIV [AM: virus responsible for aids] virus de l'immuno-déficience humaine [AM: virus responsable du sida]
humerus [AM: bone of the upper arm] humérus *m* [AM: os unique du bras]
humour humeur *f*
  ▪ aqueous/vitreous humour (of the eye) = humeur aqueuse/vitreuse; vitrée de l'œil
hump; gibbosity gibbosité *f*
hydration; moisturizing (eg of skin) hydratation *f*
hydrocephalus hydrocéphalie *f*
hydrocortisone hydrocortisone *f*

hydrogen peroxide   eau *f* oxygénée
hydronephrosis   hydronéphrose *f*
hydrotherapy   hydrothérapie *f*
hygiene   hygiène *f*
hymen   hymen *m*
hyper- (prefix); excess or increase   hyper- (préfixe); excès ou augmentation
hyperactive   hyperactif,-ive *adj*
hyperactivity   hyperactivité *f*
hypercholesterolemia   hypercholestérolemie *f*
hyperglycaemia; hyperglycemia   hyperglycémie *f*
hyperhidrosis; excess perspiration   hyperhidrose *f*
hyperparathyroidism   hyperparathyroïdie *f*
hypertension; high blood pressure   hypertension *f*
  ▪ high blood pressure = hypertension artérielle
  ▪ I have high blood pressure = je souffre d'hypertension
  ▪ intracranial hypertension = hypertension intracrânienne
hypertensive   hypertensif,-ive *adj*
hyperthermia   hyperthermie *f*
hypertrophy   hypertrophie *f*
hyperventilation   hyperventilation *f*
  ▪ to hyperventilate = être en hyperventilation
hypnosis   hypnose *f*
hypnotherapy   hypnothérapie *f*
hypnotic; sleep inducing (eg sleeping pill)   hypnotique *m*; also *adj*
hypo- (prefix); insufficiency; decrease   hypo- (préfixe); insuffisance; diminution
hypoallergenic   hypoallergénique *adj*
hypochondria   hypocondrie *f*
hypochondriac   hypocondriaque *m,f*; also *adj*; malade *m,f* imaginaire
hypodermic needle   aiguille *f* pour injections
hypodermic syringe   seringue *f* pour injections
hypoglycaemia   hypoglycémie *f*
hypotensive   hypotensif,-ive *adj*
hypothalamus   hypothalamus *m*
hypothermia   hypothermie *f*
hypothyroidism   hypothyroïdie *f*
hysterectomy   [AM: removal of uterus]   hystérectomie *f* [AM: ablation de l'utérus]
hysteria   hystérie *f*
hysteric; hysterical   hystérique *m,f*; also *adj*
hysteroscope   hystéroscope *m*
hysteroscopy   hystéroscopie *f*

I

idiocy idiotie *f*
ileitis [AM: inflammation of the ileum] iléite *f* [AM: inflammation de l'iléon]
ileum [AM: lower part of the small intestine] iléon *m* [AM: partie terminale de l'intestin grêle]
iliac iliaque *adj*
- hip bone = os iliaque
iliac artery artère *f* iliaque
ill; sick; sickness mal
- I feel sick = j'ai mal au cœur
- I have a pain here = j'ai mal ici
- it hurts = j'ai mal ici
illness; disease maladie *f*
- childhood disease ou complaint = maladie infantile; maladie d'enfant
- contagious illness/disease = maladie contagieuse
- fatal illness/disease = maladie mortelle
- infectious disease = maladie infectieuse
- legionnaires' disease = maladie du légionnaire
- mental illness = maladie mentale
- occupational disease = maladie du travail
- Parkinson's disease = maladie de Parkinson
- sexually transmitted disease, STD = maladie sexuellement transmissible
- sickness; illness; ill health = la maladie
- skin disease = maladie de peau
- sleeping sickness = maladie du sommeil
- tropical disease = maladie tropicale
- venereal disease, VD = maladie vénérienne
- wasting disease = maladie de langueur
imbecile; imbecilic imbécile *m,f*; also *adj*
imbecility; idiocy imbécillité *f*
immersion syncope hydrocution *f*
immune system système *m* immunitaire; defenses *fpl* immunitaires
immunity immunité *f*
immunization immunisation *f*
immunize (to) immuniser *v*
- to immunize against = immuniser contre
immunodeficient immunodéficitaire *adj*
immunologist immunologiste *m,f*; immunologue *m,f*
immunology immunologie *f*
impetigo impétigo *m*; gourme *f*
implant implant *m*

- dental implant = implant dentaire
implant (to) implanter *v*
impotence impotence *f*; impuissance *f*
incisor (tooth) incisive *f*; dent *f* incisive
  - lower/upper incisor = incisive inférieure/supérieure *f*
incompatible blood group incompatibilité *f* sanguine
incontinence; enuresis (urine) [AM: lack of control of passing urine or faeces]
  incontinence *f* [AM: incapacité de contrôler l'emission d'urines ou de matières fécales]
incontinence pad couche *f* pour incontinents
incontinent; enuretic incontinent,-e *adj*
incubation incubation *f*
incubation period période *f* d'incubation
incubator couveuse *f*
incurable incurable *m,f*; also *adj*
index finger; forefinger index *m*
indication indication *f*
  - remedial indication = indication thérapeutique
indigestion dyspepsie *f*; indigestion *f*
induced hypothermia hibernation *f* artificielle
industrial disease; occupational disease maladie *f* professionnelle
industrial hygiene hygiène *f* du travail
infancy petite enfance *f*; bas âge
infantile; child's; children's infantile *adj*
infarction; infarct [AM: dead tissue due to failure of blood supply] infarctus *m* [AM:
  nécrose d'un tissu à la suite d'un apport de sang insuffisant]
infect (to) infecter *v*
  - a poisoned/infected foot/finger = un pied/doigt infecté
  - it's infected = c'est infecté
  - to become infected; to become septic = s'infecter
infection infection *f*
  - you've got an infection = vous avez une infection
infectious infectieux,-ieuse *adj*
infertility infertilité *f*
infest (to) infester *v*
infestation infestation *f*
infirmity infirmité *f*
inflammation inflammation *f*; échauffement *m*
  - constipation = échauffement du ventre
inflammatory inflammatoire *adj*
influenza; flu grippe *f*
  - influenza vaccine = vaccin contre la grippe

- she has influenza = elle a la grippe
- to get or to go down with influenza = faire grippe

influx   influx *m*
- (nerve) impulse = influx nerveux

infrared radiation   rayonnement *m* infrarouge
infrared thermometer   thermomètre *m* à infrarouges
ingrowing nail   ongle *m* incarné
inhalation   inhalation *f*
inhale (to); breathe in (to)   inhaler *v*
inhaler   inhalateur *m*
- mouth inhaler = inhalateur buccal
- pocket-size inhaler = inhalateur de poche

inhibitor; inhibitory (adj)   inhibiteur *m*; inhibiteur, inhibitrice *adj*
- inhibitor of coagulation (of blood) = inhibiteur de la coagulation

inject (to)   injecter *v*
injected   injecté,-e *adj*
injection   injection *f*; infiltration *f*; piqûre *f*
- intradermic injection = injection intradermique
- intramuscular injection = injection intramusculaire
- intravenous injection = injection intraveineuse
- subcutaneous injection = injection sous-cutanée
- to have an injection = se faire faire une piqûre

injection, to give an; jab, to give a;   piquer *v*
- to have a smallpox injection = se faire piquer contre la variole

infiltration   infiltration *f*
- to have injections = se faire faire des infiltrations

injure (to); make sore (to)   blesser *v*
injure oneself (to); hurt oneself (to)   se blesser *v*
injured person; casualty; injured; wounded   blessé *m*; blessée *f*; also *adj*
- seriously/ severely injured or wounded person = blessé grave

injury   blessure *f*
inmate (eg of a mental hospital)   interné *m*; internée *f*
inoculate (to)   inoculer *v*
- to inoculate a patient against ..... = inoculer un malade contre .....

inoculation; infection   inoculation *f*
- infection = inoculation accidentelle

insect bite   piqûre *f* d'insecte
insect repellant   crème *f* contre les insectes; lotion *f* contre les insectes
insanity   folie *f*
insomnia   insomnie *f*
- I have insomnia; I can't sleep = j'ai des insomnies

insomniac insomniaque *m,f*; also *adj*
instep cou-de-pied *m*
instil (to) instiller *v*
insufficiency; inadequacy insuffisance *f*
- cardiac insufficiency = insuffisance cardiaque
- hepatic insufficiency; liver failure = insuffisance hépatique
- renal insufficiency = insuffisance rénale
- respiratory insufficiency = insuffisance respiratoire
- thyroid insufficiency = insuffisance(s) thyroïdienne(s)

insufficient; inadequate; insufficient person insuffisant,-e *adj*; insuffisant *m*
- people with respiratory insufficiency = les insuffisants respiratoires

insufflation insufflation *f*
insufflator insufflateur *m*
insulin insuline *f*
- insulin shock = choc insulinique
- insulin treatment = insulinothérapie *f*

intelligence quotient; IQ quotient *m* intellectuel; quotient d'intelligence
intensive care réanimation *f*
- intensive care unit = service de la réanimation
- to be in intensive care = être en réanimation

intensive care unit unité *f* de soins intensifs
interferon interféron *m*
intermission intermission *f*
intermittence; intermittency intermittence *f*
intern (to) (eg in a psychiatric hospital) interner *v*
internal bleeding hémorragie *f* interne
internal; interior interne *adj*
interrupt (to); break off (to); terminate (to) interrompre *v*
- to terminate a pregnancy = interrompre une grossesse

intervene (to); operate (to) intervenir *v*
- the surgeon has decided to operate = le chirurgien a décidé d'intervenir

intervention; operation intervention *f*
- he has just had a minor operation = il vient de subir une petite intervention
- surgical operation = une intervention chirurgicale

intestinal intestinal,-e *adj*
- intestinal blockage = blocage *m* intestinal

intestine intestin *m*
- bowels = intestins
- large intestine = gros intestin *m*
- small intestine; bowel = intestin *m* grêle

intraocular pressure pression *f* intraoculaire; tension *f* intraoculaire/oculaire

Intubate (to)   intuber *v*
Intubation; cannulation   intubation *f*; tubage *m*
Invalid   infirme *m,f*
Invalid; sick person; patient (eg of doctor)   malade *m,f*
  ■ hypochondriac = malade imaginaire
  ■ mentally ill person = malade mental
  ■ seriously ill person = grand malade
Invalid carriage   voiture *f* d'invalide
Inversion (of an organ)   déviation *f*
Involute   involutif,-ive *adj*
  ■ involution = processus involutif
Involution   involution *f*
Ionizing radiation   radiation *f* ionisante
Iridocyclitis   iridocyclite *f*
Iris (eye)   iris *m*
Iritis   [AM: inflammation of the iris]   iritis *m*   [AM: inflammation de l'iris]
Iron   fer *m*
Irradiation; radiation   irradiation *f*
Irreducible (eg hernia)   irréductible *adj* (par ex. hernie)
Irrigate (to)   irriguer *v*
Irrigation   irrigation *f*
Irrigator (appliance)   irrigateur *m*
Irritable bowel syndrome   syndrome *m* de l'intestin irritable; colopathie *f*
  fonctionnelle
Irritable colon   côlon *m* irritable
Irritant   irritant *m*; irritant,-e *adj*
Irritation   irritation *f* (syn. excitation)
Isolation   isolement *m*
  ■ isolation hospital = hôpital d'isolement
Itch (to)   démanger *v*
  ■ my arm is itching = ça me démange au bras
  ■ my back is itching = le dos me démange
Itch; itching   démangeaison *f*; prurit *m*
  ■ my back/foot is itching = j'ai des démangeaisons dans le dos/dans le pied
  ■ to be itching = avoir des démangeaisons
Itching; pruritus   prurit *m*

J,K

jaundice; icterus jaunisse *f*; ictère *m*
jaw mâchoire *f*
- lower/upper jaw = mâchoire inférieure/supérieure
jaw surgery chirurgie *f* maxillaire
jawbone; maxilla maxillaire *m*
- lower/upper jawbone = maxillaire inférieur/supérieur
jejunum [AM: part of small intestine] jéjunum *m* [AM: partie de l'intestin grêle]
jogging jogging *m*
- to go for one's daily jog = faire son jogging quotidien
- to go jogging = aller faire un jogging
joint articulation *f*
joint blocking blocage *m* articulaire
juvenile rheumatoid arthritis arthrite chronique juvénile; maladie de Still
Kaposi's sarcoma sarcome de Kaposi
keratin kératine *f*
keratitis [AM: inflammation of the cornea] kératite *f* [AM: inflammation de la cornée]
kidney rein *m*
- kidney stone = calcul rénal
- right/left kidney = rein droit/gauche
- to have (a) backache = avoir mal aux reins
kleptomania kleptomanie *f*
knee genou *m*
- my knee is dislocated = mon genou s'est déboîté
knee support (bandage or plaster) genouillère *f* (bandage ou plâtre)

L

L-dopa [AM: used in treatment of Parkinson's disease] L-dopa *f* [AM: utilisée dans le traitement de la maladie de Parkinson]
laboratory laboratoire *m*
labour (childbirth) travail *m*
- labour ward = salle de travail
- to go into/start labour = entrer en travail
- woman in labour = femme en travail
labour room chambre *f* de travail préparatoire à l'acouchement
lachrymal apparatus appareil *m* lacrymal

lachrymal caruncle   caroncule *f* lacrymale
lachrymal ducts; lachrymatory ducts   conduits *mpl* lacrymaux
lachrymatory glands   glandes *fpl* lacrymales
lack of coordination; incoordination   incoordination *f*
lactation   lactation *f*
lance (to); burst (to) (eg abcess, boil)   percer *v*
lancet   lancette *f*
lanolin   lanoline *f* (graisse de laine)
laparotomy   [AM: opening the abdominal cavity]   laparotomie *f* [AM: ouverture de la cavité abdominale]
laryngectomy   [AM: removal of part or whole of larynx]   laryngectomie *f* [AM: ablation de la totalité ou une partie du larynx]
laryngitis   [AM: inflammation of the larynx]   laryngite *f* [AM: inflammation du larynx]
laryngoscope   laryngoscope *m*
laryngoscopy   [AM: visual examination of larynx using a laryngoscope]   laryngoscopie *f* [AM: examen visuel du larynx à l'aide d'un laryngoscope]
larynx   larynx *m*
laser   laser *m*
Lassa fever   fièvre *f* de Lassa
lassitude   lassitude *f*
latency time   temps *m* de latence
laxative   laxatif *m*; laxatif,-ive *adj*
lead poisoning; plumbism; saturnism   saturnisme *m*
lead poisoning colic   coliques *fpl* de plomb
leg   jambe *f*
  ▪ articulated leg = jambe articulée
  ▪ artificial leg = jambe artificielle
legionnaires' disease   pneumonie *f* des légionnaires
leprosy   lèpre *f*
lesbian   lesbienne *f*; also *adj*
lesbianism   lesbianisme *m*
lesion   lésion *f*
  ▪ internal injuries = lésions internes
  ▪ pulmonary lesion = lésion pulmonaire
lethargy   léthargie *f*
leucocyte   [AM: white blood cell]   leucocyte *m* [AM: globule blanc]
leucotomy   leucotomie *f*; lobotomie *f* cérébrale
leukaemia; leukemia   leucémie *f*
leukoma; leucoma   [AM: corneal opacity]   taie *f* [AM: opacité de la cornée]
leukorrhea; leucorrhea   leucorrhée *f*; pertes *fpl* blanches
libido   libido *f*
life expectancy   espérance *f* de vie

ligament ligament *m*
ligature ligature *f*
ligature (to); tie up (to) ligaturer *v*
limb membre *m*
- upper/lower limbs = membres supérieurs/inférieurs
lip lèvre *f*
- corners of the lips/mouth = commissures des lèvres
- the edges of a wound/incision = les lèvres d'une plaie/incision
- upper/lower lip = lèvre supérieure/inférieure
lip gloss brillant *m* à lèvres
lip liner; lip pencil crayon *m* à lèvres
lip salve pommade *f* pour les lèvres; pommade *f* rosat
lipid lipide *m*
liposoluble; fat soluble liposoluble *adj*
liposuction liposuccion *f*
lipstick rouge *m* à lèvres
listeriosis; listeria listériose *f*
little finger auriculaire *m*
liver foie *m*
- abscess of the liver = abcès du foie
- cancer of the liver = cancer du foie
lobe, lower (lung) lobe *m* inférieur
lobe, middle (lung) lobe *m* moyen
lobe, upper (lung) lobe *m* supérieur
lobule; ear lobe lobule *m*
locomotor ataxia ataxie *f* locomotrice
locum; replacement remplaçant *m*; remplaçante *f*
longevity longévité *f*
lordosis lordose *f*
lose weight (to) mincir *v*
- slimming diet = régime pour mincir
loss; losing (eg blood) perte *f*
- heavy bleeding = pertes de sang
- loss of consciousness, fainting = perte de connaissance
- loss of memory, memory loss = perte de mémoire
- vaginal discharge, leucorrhœa = pertes blanches
louse; lice *(pl)*; pediculus pou *m*; poux *mpl*
- to have lice = avoir des poux
low blood pressure hypotension *f* artérielle
low-calorie dishes cuisine *f* minceur
lower teeth dents *fpl* du bas

lumbago lombalgie *f*; lumbago *m*
lumbar lombaire *adj*
- in the lumbar region = dans la région lombaire
lumbar puncture ponction *f* lombaire
lump (tumour) grosseur *f*
- to have a lump in the breast = avoir un grosseur au sein
lump; bump bosse *f*
lunacy folie *f*; démence *f*
lung poumon *m*
- an abscess of the lung = abcés du poumon
- left/right lung = poumon gauche/droit
lupus (vulgaris) lupus *m* (vulgaire)
lymph lymphe *f*
lymph node; lymph gland ganglion *m* lymphatique
lymph vessel vaisseau *m* lymphatique
lymphangitis lymphangite *f*
lymphatic lymphatique *adj*
- lymphatic system = système *m* lymphatique
lymphatic drainage drainage *m* lymphatique
lymphosarcoma lymphosarcome *m*

M

macula (discolouration spot) macule *f*
macula degeneration dégénérescence *f* maculaire
mad cow disease maladie *f* de la vache folle
madness; lunacy; insanity folie *f*
magnesium magnésium *m*
magnifying glass loupe *f*
make-up (cosmet) fard *m*
- blusher = fard à joues
- eye-shadow = fard à paupières
make-up (to) maquiller *v*
make-up; making-up maquillage *m*
make-up pencil crayon *m* de maquillage
make-up remover démaquillant *m*
malaria malaria *f*; paludisme *m*; fièvre *f* paludéenne
malaria stricken impaludé,-e *adj*

malarial paludéen,-enne *adj*; malarien,-ienne *adj*
male menopause; male climacteric andropause *f*
malignancy malignité *f*
malignant malin, maligne *adj* (ant. bénin, bénigne)
  ▪ malignant tumour = tumeur maligne
malnutrition sous-alimentation *f*
mammary mammaire *adj*
  ▪ mammary abscess = abcès mammaire
  ▪ mammary glands = glandes mammaires
mammography [AM: radiographic examination of the breasts] mammographie *f*,
  mastographie *f* [AM: examen des seins par radiographie]
mammogram mammographie *f*
mania manie *f*
manicure manucure *f*
  ▪ to manicure one's nails = se faire les ongles
manicure set tousse *f* de manucure
manipulation manipulation *f*
  ▪ genetically engineered = obtenu par manipulation génétique
  ▪ manipulation of the spine = manipulation vertébrale
marasmus [AM: nutritional deficiency leading to progressive emaciation] marasme *m* [AM:
  carence nutritionnelle menant à l'emaciation progressive]
marker marqueur *m*
marrow moelle *f*
  ▪ bone marrow = moelle osseuse
  ▪ bone marrow transplant = greffe de moelle osseuse
mascara mascara *m*
mask; face-pack masque *m*
  ▪ oxygen mask = masque à oxygène
massage massage *m*
  ▪ cardiac massage = massage cardiaque
massage (to); mass (to) masser *v*
  ▪ to have a massage = se faire masser
masseur; masseuse masseur *m*; masseuse *f*
mastectomy [AM: removal of mammary gland] mastectomie *f* [AM: ablation de la glande
  mammaire]
mastitis mastite *f*
mastoid mastoïde *f*, also *adj*
  ▪ mastoid process (protuberance) = apophyse *f* mastoïde
mastoiditis mastoïdite *f*
maternity department; obstetric department service *m* d'accouchement; service
  m de maternité; département *m* de maternité
matter matière *f*

163

medulla

- faecal matter; faeces = matières fécales

mattress   matelas *m*
- air mattress; air bed = matelas pneumatique
- water mattress = matelas à eau

maturation   maturation *f*

maxillary   maxillaire *adj*

measles   rougeole *f*

measure (to); measure out (to)   doser *v*

medical care; health care.   soins *mpl* médicaux

medical certificate   certificat *m* médical; attestation *f* médicale

medical consultant   chef *m* de service

medical dossier   dossier *m* médical

medical examination   examen *m* médical

medical fees   honoraires *mpl* médicaux

medical law   droit *m* médical

medical registration card (France)   carte *f* vitale

medical student; medic (slang)   carabin *m* (argot)

medical supervision   surveillance *f* médicale

medically degenerate person; degenerate (adj)   dégénéré *m*; dégénérée *f*; also *adj*

medicine   médecine *f*
- alternative medicine = médecine alternative/douce/naturelle
- alternative medicine = médecines douces/parallèles
- casualty (department) = médecine d'urgence (service)
- complementary medicine = médecine parallèle
- emergency treatment = médecine d'urgence
- general medicine = médecine générale
- natural medicine = médecine naturelle
- occupational or industrial medicine = médecine du travail
- paediatrics = médecine infantile
- preventive medicine = médecine préventive
- remedial medicine = médecine curative

medicine; drug; remedy; cure   médicament *m*; remède *m*; agent *m* thérapeutique
- conventional medicine/remedy = médicament allopathique
- homeopathic medicine/remedy = médicament homéopathique
- I am taking this medicine = je prends ce médicament
- is it safe to give to children? = c'est sans danger pour les enfants?
- over-the-counter remedy = médicament de confort

meditation   méditation *f*

medulla   moelle *f*

megalomania mégalomanie *f*
melancholia mélancolie *f*
melanin mélanine *m*
melanism mélanisme *m*
melanoma mélanome *m*
membrane membrane *f*
 ■ little membrane = membranule *f*
membrane (skin) (of blood clot) couenne *f*
 ■ buffy coat = couenne inflammatoire
Ménière's disease vertige *m* de Ménière; maladie *f* de Ménière
memory memoire *f*
meninges méninges *mpl*
meningitis méningite *f*
 ■ meningococcus (micro-organism) = méningocoque
menopausal ménopausée *adj*
menopause ménopause *f*
menorrhagia ménorragie *f*
menses menstruation *f*; règles *fpl*
menstrual menstruel,-elle *adj*
menstruation menstruation *f*
mental age âge *m* mental
mental deficiency déficience *f* mentale; débilité *f* mentale; faiblesse *f* mentale
mental health santé *f* mentale
mental illness maladie *f* mentale
mental retardation déficience *f* intellectuelle
mentally ill person malade *m,f* mental
mercury mercure *m*
metabolism métabolisme *m*
metacarpals os *mpl* du métacarpe
metacarpus métacarpe *m*
metatarsus métatarse *m*
 ■ metatarsals = os du métatarse
method méthode *f*
methylene blue [AM: blue dye used as antiseptic] bleu *m* de méthylène [AM: colorant bleu utilisé comme antiseptique]
microbe; germ microbe *m*
microbiologist microbiologiste *m,f*
microbiology microbiologie *f*
micturition miction *f*
middle finger majeur *m*

165

muscle

- to be over 18 = être majeure
middle-aged entre deux âges
midwife; obstetrician accoucheuse *f*; accoucheur *m*; sage-femme *f*
midwifery; obstetrics obstétrique *f*
migraine; sick headache migraine *f*
minipill minipilule *f*
minoxidil [AM: vasodilator drug] minoxidil *m* [AM: médicament ayant propriétés vasodilatatrices]
miscarriage fausse couche *f*; avortement *m* spontané
- to have a miscarriage = faire une fausse couche
mixed feeding allaitement *m* mixte
moisturising face-pack masque *m* hydratant
molar (tooth) molaire *f*
mole; beauty spot grain *m* de beauté; lentigo *m*
monitoring monitorage *m*; monitoring *m*
morbid morbide *adj*
morning-after pill pilule *f* du lendemain
morning sickness nausée *f* (du matin); nausées *fpl* matinales
morphine morphine *f*
mosquito repellent produit *m* antimoustique
motor neuron neurone *m* moteur
mouth bouche *f*
- mouth to mouth resuscitation = bouche-à-bouche *m*
- open your mouth; put your tongue out = ouvrez la bouche; tirez la langue
mouth ulcer; aphta aphte *m*
mouthwash eau *f* dentifrice
mucous muqueux,-euse *adj*; glaireux,-euse *adj*
mucous membrane muqueuse *f*
mucoviscidosis [AM: fibrocystic disease of the pancreas] mucoviscidose *f* [AM: maladie fibrose kystique du pancréas]
mucus glaire *f*
- cervical mucus = glaire cervicale
- to have catarrh = avoir des glaires
mud bath bain *m* de boue
multiple (eg fractures) multiple *adj*
mumps, the les oreillons *mpl*
muscle muscle *m*
- abdominal muscles = abdominaux *mpl*
- abductor muscle = abducteur *m*; also *adj*
- adductor muscle = adducteur *m* ; also *adj*

- biceps brachial muscle = muscle biceps brachial
- biceps femoris muscle = muscle biceps crural
- deltoid; deltoidal muscle = deltoïde *m*; deltoïde *adj*
- extensor muscle = extenseur *m*; also *adj*
- flexor muscle = fléchisseur *m*; also *adj*
- gluteal muscles = muscles *mpl* fessiers
- iliopsoas muscle = psoas *m*; muscle psoas-iliaque
- pectoralis major muscle = muscle grand pectoral
- quadripeds femoris muscle = muscle quadriceps crural
- rotator muscle = rotateur *m*; also *adj*
- strained or pulled muscle = élongation *f*
- to strain or pull a calf muscle = se faire une élongation au mollet

muscular musculaire *adj*
musculature musculature *f*
mutagen mutagène
muteness mutité *f*; mutisme *m*
myasthenia gravis myasthénie *f*
mycosis ; fungus disease mycose *f*
- athlete's foot = mycose du pied
- vaginal thrush = mycose vaginale

mycotoxicosis mycotoxicose *f*
mycotoxin mycotoxine *f*
myelitis myélite *f*
myocarditis myocardite *f*
myocardium myocarde *m*
myoglobin myoglobine *f*
myopathy myopathie *f*
myopia myopie *f*
myxoedema; myxedema myxœdème *m*

N

nail clippers coupe-ongles *m*; pince *f* à ongles
nail scissors ciseaux *mpl* à ongles
nail varnish remover/solvent dissolvant *m*
nail varnish; nail polish vernis *m* à ongles
nailbrush brosse *f* à ongles
nailfile lime *f* à ongles

neuralgic

nails ongles *mpl*
nape (of the neck) nuque *f*
nappy; diaper couche *f* pour bébés
- disposable nappy/diaper = couche jetable
- disposable nappy/diaper = couche-culotte *f*
- disposable nappy/diaper = couche en cellulose
nappy rash érythème *m* fessier
- to have nappy rash = avoir les fesses irritées
narcosis narcose *f*
nasal nasal,-e *adj*
nasal cavity cavité *f* nasale
nausea; sick nausée *f*
- I feel sick/nauseous = j'ai la nausée
navel; umbilicus nombril *m*; ombilic *m*
neck cou *m*
necrosis nécrose *f*
needle (eg of syringe) aiguille *f*
nephritic lithiasis lithiase *f* rénale
nephritis; acute Bright's disease [AM: inflammation of the kidney] néphrite *f* [AM: inflammation du rein]
nephrosis néphrose *f*
nerve nerf *m*
- cranial nerves = nerfs *mpl* crâniens
- motor nerve = nerf moteur
- ophthalmic nerve nerf ophtalmique
- optic nerve = nerf optique
- phrenic nerve = nerf phrènique
- pneumogastric nerve (vagus nerve) = nerf pneumogastrique *f*
- sensory nerve = nerf sensitif
- spinal nerves = nerfs *mpl* spinaux
- vagus nerve = nerf vague
nervous nerveux, nerveuse *adj*
- false pregnancy; phantom pregnancy = grossesse nerveuse
- nervous breakdown = dépression nerveuse
- nervous system = système nerveux
nervousness; nervous tension nervosité *f*
nettle rash; urticaria; hives urticaire *f*
neural neural,-e *adj*
neuralgia névralgie *f*
neuralgic névralgique *adj*
- nerve centre = centre/point névralgique

neurasthenia; depression neurasthénie *f*
neurasthenic; depressed neurasthénique *adj*
neuritis névrite *f*
neuroleptic neuroleptique *m*; also *adj*
neurological neurologique *adj*
neurologist neurologue *m,f*
neurology [AM: study and treatment of the nervous system] neurologie *f* [AM: étude et traitement du système nerveux]
neuroma [AM: tumour] névrome *m* [AM: tumeur]
neuron neurone *m*
neuronal neuronal,-e *adj*
neurosis névrose *f*
  ▪ obsessional/phobic neurosis = névrose obsessionnelle/phobique
neurotic névrotique *adj*
neutralise (to); block (to) (pain) neutraliser *v*
nevus; naevus; birthmark; angioma nævus *m*
new-born baby nouveau-né,-e *m,f*; also *adj*
new-born baby; (unweaned) infant nourrisson *m*
nicotine patch patch *m* à la nicotine
nightmare cauchmar *m*
nipple mamelon *m*
nodule nodule *m*
noradrenaline noradrénaline *f*
normal normal,-e *adj*
nose nez *m*
  ▪ to have a blocked nose = avoir le nez bouché
nose drops gouttes *fpl* pour le nez
nosebleed saignement *m* de nez
nostril narine *f*
nourishing; nutritive nutritif,-ive *adj*
nuclear magnetic resonance imaging imagerie *f* par résonance magnétique; I.R.M.
nucleus noyau *m*
numbness engourdissement *m*
numeration numération *f*
  ▪ blood count = numération globulaire
nurse (female) infirmière *f*
nurse (male) infirmier *m*
nurse, district infirmière *f* visiteuse/visitante
nurse, home garde-malade *m,f*
nurse, head/chief infirmière *f* en chef

nurse, head; charge nurse surveillant *m*; surveillante *f*
nurse, registered; nurse with diploma infirmière *f* diplômée
nurse, visiting infirmière *f* visiteuse/visitante
nursing auxiliary; nurse's aide aide-soignant,-e *m,f*
nutrition nutrition *f*
nystagmus nystagmus *m*

O

obese obèse *adj*
obesity obésité *f*
observation observation *f*
- to be/to put under observation = être/mettre en observation
obstetric obstétrique *adj*
- obstetric clinic = clinique obstétrique
obstetric department; maternity department service *m* d'obstétrique
obstetrician médecin *m* accoucheur; obstétricien *m*; obstétricienne *f*
obstruct (to) (eg an artery) oblitérer *v*
obstruction (eg of a cavity); choking up (of hernia) engouement *m*
obstruction; blockage obstruction *f*
occipital occipital,-e *adj*
- occipital region/area = région occipital
occiput occiput *m*
occlude (to) occlure *v*
occlusion occlusion *f*
- intestinal blockage = occlusion intestinale
occupational disease maladie *f* du travail
occupational therapy ergothérapie *f*; thérapeutique *f* occupationnelle
oculist; ophthalmologist oculiste *m*
- I am looking for an optician = je cherche un oculiste
oedema œdème *m*
Oedipus complex œdipe, complex d'
oesophagus; esophagus; gullet œsophage *m*
oestrogen (female hormone) œstrogène *m*
oil huile *f*
- castor oil = huile de ricin
- cod liver oil = huile de foie de morue
- essential oil = huile essentielle

- evening primrose oil = huile d'onagre
- olive oil = huile d'olive
- sunflower oil = huile de tournesol
- wheat germ oil = huile de germe de blé

ointment pommade *f*
- ointment for burns = pommade contre les brûlures
- ointment for haemorrhoids = remède *m* hémorroïdaire

old age vieillesse *f*
olfaction olfaction *f*
oliguria oligurie *f*
operate (to) opérer *v*
- he had an operation for a tumour/ to remove a tumour = on l'a opéré d'une tumeur
- to have an operation = se faire opérer
- to have one's tonsils removed = se faire opérer des amygdales
- we'll have to operate = nous devons opérer
- will he need an operation? = il faudra l'opérer
- you will need an operation = il va falloir opérer

operating (eg methods) opératoire *adj*
- post-operative depression = dépression opératoire
- post-operative illness = maladie opératoire

operating theatre; operating room théâtre *m* d'opérations; salle *f* d'opérations
operation opération *f*
ophthalmia [AM: eye inflammation] ophtalmie *f* [AM: inflammation de l'œil]
ophthalmologist ophtalmologiste *m*; ophtalmologue *m*
ophthalmoscope ophtalmoscope *m*
ophthalmoscopy ophtalmoscopie *f*
opthalmology ophtalmologie *f*
optician opticien *m*
oral oral,-e *adj*
oral cavity cavité *f* buccale
oral medication; throat preparation or spray collutoire *m*
orally oralement adv
orbit; eye socket orbite *f*
orchitis orchite *f*
organ organe *m*
- digestive organs = organes digestifs
- external/internal genital organs = organes génitaux externes/internes

organism organisme *m*
orthodontics orthodontie *f*
orthopaedic surgeon orthopédiste *m,f*; chirurgien *m*/chirurgienne *f* orthopédiste

orthopaedic; orthopedic orthopédique *adj*
- orthopaedic surgery = chirurgie *f* orthopédique

orthopedics orthopédie *f*

Osgood-Schlatter disease Osgood-Schlatter, maladie d'

ossification ossification *f*

osteitis ostéite *f*

osteoarthritis;degenerative joint disease ostéoarthrite *f*, arthrose *f*
- osteoarthritis of the knee = arthrose du genou

osteomyelitis ostéomyélite *f*

osteopath ostéopathe *m,f*

osteopathy ostéopathie *f*

osteoporosis ostéoporose *f*

osteosarcoma ostéosarcome *m*

osteosclerosis ostéosclérose *f*

otitis otite *f*

otology [AM: study of diseases of the ear] otologie *f* [AM: étude des maladies de l'oreille]

otorhinolaryngology oto-rhino-laryngologie *f*

ovary ovaire *m*

overdosage; excess dose surdosage *m*

overdose (eg drug) overdose *f*

overdose; excess dose surdose *f*

overheat échauffer *v*
- I'm a bit constipated = je suis un peu échauffé
- to inflame the skin = échauffer la peau
- to overheat the blood = échauffer le sang

overheating échauffement *m*

overweight; excess weight surpoids *m*

ovulate (to) ovuler *v*

ovulation ovulation *f*

ovum ovule *m*

oxygen oxygène *m*
- oxgen cylinder; oxygen bottle = bouteille d'oxygène

oxygen tent tente *f* à oxygène

oxygen therapy oxygénothérapie *f*

P

pacemaker pacemaker *m*; stimulateur *m* cardiaque; stimulateur *m* artificiel

pacifier; dummy sucette *f*
pack enveloppement *m*
- cold pack = enveloppement froid
- ice-pack = enveloppement glacé
pack with gauze (to) mécher *v*
pack; dressing mèche *f*
paediatric nurse puéricultrice *f*
paediatrician; pediatrician pédiatre *m,f*
paediatrics; pediatrics pédiatrie *f*
paedology; pedology pédologie *f*
Paget's disease of bone Paget, maladie *f* osseuse de
Paget's disease; Paget's carcinoma (of nipple) maladie *f* cutanée de Paget
pain (see also ache) douleur *f*; mal *m*
- I have a pain in my arm = j'ai mal au bras
- sharp pain; shooting pain = élancement *m*
- to be in pain = souffrir; avoir mal
pain relieving antidouleur *adj*
painful; aching douloureux,-euse *adj*
painkiller; analgesic calmant *m* analgésique
palate palais *m*
- cleft palate = palais fendu
palliative palliatif *m*; palliatif,-ive *adj*
pallor; paleness pâleur *f*
palm paume *f*
palpate (to) palper *v*
palpation palpation *f*; palper *m*
palpitations palpitations *fpl*
palsy; paralysis paralysie *f*
- shaking palsy = paralysie agitante
paludal (relating to malaria) paludéen,-enne; paludique; palustre *adj*
pancreas pancréas *m*
pancreatic pancréatique *adj*
pancreatitis pancreatite *f*
panic attack attaque de panique
panty liner protège-slip *m*
papule papule *f*
papulo-pustule papulo-pustule *f*
paracetamol [AM: analgesic and antipyretic] paracétamol *m* [AM: analgésique et antipyrétique]
paralyse (to); paralyze (to) paralyser *v*
paralysis paralysie *f*

- facial paralysis = paralysie faciale
- infantile paralysis; poliomyelitis = paralysie infantile

paralytic; paralysed man, woman   paralysé *m*; paralysée *f*
paramedical   paramédical,-e *adj*
paranoïa   paranoïa *f*
paraphimosis   paraphimosis *m*
paraplegia   paraplégie *f*
paraplegic   paraplégique *m,f*, also *adj*
parasite   parasite *m*
parasitic   parasitique *adj*; parisitaire *adj*
parasympathetic nervous system   système *m* parasympathique
parathyroid; parathyroid gland   parathyroïde *f*
paratyphoid fever   paratyphoïde *f*; fièvre *f* paratyphoïde
paresis; partial paralysis   parésie *f*
Parkinson's disease   maladie de Parkinson
parotiditis   parotidite *f*
paroxysm   paroxysme *m*
pass (to); exceed (to)   dépasser *v*
  - do not exceed the prescribed dose = ne pas dépasser la dose prescrite
pass on (to) (an illness)   communiquer *v* (une maladie)
patch-test   patch-test *m*
patella; kneecap   rotule *f*
pathogenic   pathogène *adj*
  - pathogen = agent pathogène
pathological   pathologique *adj*
pathological laboratory   laboratoire *m* pathologique
pathologist   pathologiste *m,f*
pathology   pathologie *f*
patient   patient *m*; patiente *f*
patient (who has had an operation)   opéré *m*; opérée *f*
pectoral; chest   pectoral,-e *adj*
  - cough syrup = sirop pectoral
  - pectoral muscles = muscles pectoraux
pedal artery   artère *f* pédieuse
pediculosis; infestation with lice   pédiculose *f*
pellagra   pellagre *f*
pelvis   bassin *m*; pelvis *m*
  - lower pelvis = petit bassin
penicillin   pénicilline *f*
  - I am allergic to penicillin = je suis allergique à la pénicilline
penis   pénis *m*; verge *f*

pepsin pepsine *f*
peptic ulcer ulcère *m* de l'estomac; ulcère *m* gastro-duodénal
percuss (to) percuter *v*
percussion; percussion massage percussion *f*
percutaneous percutané,-e *adj*
perforate (to) perforer *v*
perforation perforation *f*
perforator perforateur *m*
perfume; scent parfum *m*
periadontitis parodontite *f*
periarthritis périarthrite *f*
pericarditis péricardite *f*
pericardium péricarde *m*
perineum périnée *m*
period of hallucination bouffée *f* délirante
period; menstruation règles *fpl*
  ▪ I haven't had my period for three months = je n'ai pas eu mes règles depuis trois mois
  ▪ I have period pains = j'ai des règles douloureuses
peristalsis péristaltisme *m*
peritonitis péritonite *f*
peritonium péritoine *m*
perleche [AM: inflammation of the corners of the lips] perlèche *f* [AM: inflammation des commissures des lèvres]
pernicious pernicieux,-ieuse *adj*
peroxide peroxyde *m*
  ▪ hydrogen peroxide = eau oxygénée
person who suffers from a liver complaint hépatique *m,f*
person with Down's syndrome mongolien *m*; mongolienne *f*
personality test test *m* de personnalité
perspiration; sweat perspiration *f*; sueur *f*; transpiration *f*
pessary pessaire *m*
pessary; vaginal suppository ovule *m*
  ▪ antifungus pessary = ovule antifongique
petit mal; minor epilepsy petit mal *m* épileptique
petrissage; kneading massage pétrissage *m*
  ▪ to knead = pétrir *v*
phalanx (phalanges *pl*) (finger bone) phalange *f*
pharmacist pharmacien *m*; pharmacienne *f*
pharmacology pharmacologie *f*
pharyngitis pharyngite *f*

175

pharynx pharynx *m*
phase; stage phase *f*
phlebitis phlébite *f*
phlegm mucosité *f*; glaire *f*
phobia phobie *f*
phosphorus phosphore *m*
photophobia [AM: aversion to light] photophobie *f* [AM: crainte de la lumière]
photosensitization photosensibilisation *f*
physical examination examen *m* fonctionel
physical rehabilitation réadaptation *f* physique
physio; physiotherapist kiné *m,f*; kinésithérapeute *m,f*
physiological laboratory laboratoire *m* physiologique
physiology physiologie *f*
physiotherapist physiothérapeute *m,f*; kinésithérapeute *m,f*
physiotherapy kinésithérapie *f*; physiothérapie *f*
phytotherapy phytothérapie *f*
pigmentation pigmentation *f*
piles hémorroïdes *fpl*
pill pilule *f*; comprimé *m*; cachet *m*; la pilule contraceptive
pill, sugar-coated dragée *f*
pimple bouton *m*
pimply bouttonneux,-euse *adj*
pin (surgical) broche *f*
pin, safety épingle *f* de sûreté
pinch mark; blood blister pinçon *m*
pinch (to) pincer *v*
pinch; pinching massage pincement *m*
pinning (eg a fractured bone) brochage *m*
pins and needles in the hands/legs (to have) fourmis *fpl* dans les mains/jambes (avoir des)
pinworm; threadworm; seatworm; oxyurid oxyure *m*
pituitary gland glande *f* pituitaire; hypophyse *f*
placebo placebo *m*
placenta; afterbirth placenta *m*
plague peste *f*
plasma bank banque *f* de plasma
plaster plâtre *m*
 ▪ to put/set in plaster = mettre dans le plâtre
plaster; sticking plaster emplâtre *m*
 ▪ **emplâtre pour les cors** = corn plaster
plastic surgeon chirurgien *m* plastique; chirurgienne *f* plastique

plastic surgery chirurgie *f* plastique
plastic surgery of the breast mammoplastie *f*, mastoplastie *f*, plastie *f* mammaire
pleura plèvre *f*
pleural cavity cavité *f* pleurale
pleurisy pleurésie *f*
pleuritic pleurétique *adj*
plexus plexus *m*
pneumococcus pneumocoque *m*
pneumoconiosis pneumoconiose *f*
pneumonia pneumonie *f* (syn. fluxion de poitrine)
 ▪ viral pneumonia = pneumonie virale
point; place; spot point *m*
 ▪ blackhead (face) = comédon *m*; point *m* noir (visage)
 ▪ nerve centre = point névralgique
 ▪ stitch = point de suture
 ▪ to have a stitch in one's side = avoir un point de côté
 ▪ to have a twinge (of pain) in one's back = avoir un point dans le dos
 ▪ to put stitches in; to stitch up = faire des points de suture à
 ▪ you have a spot of congestion there = vous avez un point de congestion là
point; tip pointe *f*
poison poison *m*
poison (to) empoisonner *v*; intoxiquer *v*
poison centre centre *m* anti-poison
poisoning empoisonnement *m*; intoxication *f*
poliomyelitis poliomyélite *f*
pollution pollution *f*
 ▪ wet dreams; nocturnal emissions = pollutions nocturnes
polyarthritis polyarthrite *f*
polymyositis polymyosite *f*
polyneuritis polynévrite *f*
polyp; polypus polype *m*
polyvalent (eg serum, vaccine) polyvalent,-e *adj*
porphyria porphyrie *f*
post-operative post-opératoire *adj*
posture posture *f*
potassium potassium *m*
Pott's disease mal *m* de Pott
poultice; cataplasm cataplasme *m*
 ▪ linseed meal poultice = cataplasme de farine de lin
 ▪ mustard poultice = cataplasme de moutarde

177

- mustard poultice; mustard plaster = cataplasme sinapisé

powder   poudre *f*
  - baby powder = talc *m*
  - face powder = poudre de riz
  - tooth powder = poudre dentifrice

powder compact   poudrier *m*

powder puff   houppe *f* (à poudrer); houppette *f* (à poudrer)

practise (to); carry out (to)   pratiquer *v*

practitioner   praticien *m*; praticienne *f*

pre-eclampsia   prééclampsie *f*

pre-shave lotion   lotion *f* avant-rasage; lotion *f* pré-rasage

pregnancy   grossesse *f*
  - ectopic pregnancy = grossesse extra-utérine
  - phantom pregnancy = grossesse nerveuse
  - pregnancy test = test *m* de grossesse

pregnant   enceinte *adj*
  - I am pregnant = je suis enceinte
  - since when have you been pregnant? = depuis combien de temps êtes-vous enceinte?
  - to be pregnant with twins = être enceinte de jumeaux
  - to be three months pregnant = être enceinte de trois mois

premature (baby)   prématuré *m*; prématuré,-e *adj*

premenstrual tension; PMT   syndrome *m* prémenstruel; PMS

prenatal cliniic   clinique *f* prénatale

preoperative   préopératoire *adj*

prepuce   prépuce *m*

presbyopia; longsightedness   presbytie *f*

preschool age   âge préscolaire

prescribe (to)   ordonner *v*; prescrire *v*
  - do not exceed the prescribed dose = ne pas dépasser la dose prescrite

prescription   ordonnance *f*
  - available on prescription only = délivré uniquement sur ordonnance
  - can I get it without a prescription? = puis-je l'obtenir sans ordonnance?
  - over-the-counter medicine = médicament vendu sans ordonnance

prescription; directions   prescription *f*
  - to be taken in accordance with doctors' instructions = se conformer aux prescriptions du medecin

presence of alcohol in the blood   alcoolémie *f*
  - checking for alcohol in the blood = contrôle d'alcoolémie
  - level of alcohol in the blood = taux d'alcoolémie

present (to)   présenter *v*

presentation présentation *f*
- head/breech presentation (of baby) = présentation par la tête/le siège

pressure pression *f*
- blood pressure = pression artérielle
- pressure massage = pressions

prevention prévention *f*
preventive medicine médecine *f* préventive
priapism priapisme *m*
primary primaire *adj*
private bed lit *m* privé
probe (to) sonder *v*
probe sonde *f*
probing; probe sondage *m*
progesterone progestérone *f*
prognosis pronostic *m*
progressive évolutif,-ive *adj*
prolapse prolapsus *m*
prophylaxis prophylaxie *f*
prostaglandin prostaglandine *f*
prostate prostate *f*
- prostate cancer = cancer de la prostate

prostatectomy [AM: partial or total removal of the prostate]   prostatectomie *f* [AM: ablation partielle ou totale de la prostate]
prostatitis prostatite *f*
prosthesis prothèse *f*
prostration prostration *f*
protein proteine *f*
protuberance éminence *f*
pruritus; itching prurit *m*
pschotherapy psychothérapie *f*
psittacosis [AM: infection transmitted by birds (budgerigar, parrot]   psittacose *f* [AM: maladie transmise par les oiseaux (perruche, perroquet)]
psoriasis [AM: skin disease]   psoriasis *m*   [AM: maladie cutanée]
psychiatric psychiatrique *adj*
psychiatrist psychiatre *m,f*
psychiatry psychiatrie *f*
psychoanalysis psychanalyse *f*
psychological psychologique *adj*
psychological test test *m* psychologique
psychologist psychologue *m,f*
psychology psychologie *f*

psychopath psychopathe *m,f*, also *adj*
psychopathy psychopathie *f*
psychosis psychose *f*
puberty puberté *f*
pubic pubien,-ienne *adj*
pubis pubis *m*
- pubic hair = poils *mpl* du pubis
public health santé *f* publique
puerperal puerpéral,-e *adj*
puerperal fever fièvre *f* puerpérale
pulmonary pulmonaire *adj*
pulp cavity (tooth) cavité *f* pulpaire
pulsation; beat (eg heart) pulsation *f*
- the normal heart beat varies from 60-100 beats/minute = le rythme cardiaque normal varie de 60-100 pulsations/minute
pulse pouls *m*
- the pulse rate is about 70 beats a minute = le rhythme du pouls est d'environ 70 battements à la minute
- to take someone's pulse = prendre le pouls de quelqu'un
pulverization pulvérisation *f*
- the doctor prescribed a nasal spray = le médecin a ordonné des pulvérisations (nasales)
puncture ponction *f*
pupil (eye) pupille *f*
purgation; purgative purgation *f*
purgative purgatif *m*; purgatif,-ive *adj*
purgative; purge purge *f* (colloq)
purge (to) purger *v*
purification épuration *f*
purpura purpura *m*
pus pus *m*
pustule pustule *f*
pustulosis pustulose *f*
put on weight (to); increase (to) grossir *v*
put under stress (to) stresser *v*
- to be stressed; to be on edge = être stressé
pylorus pylore *m*
pyorrhea pyorrhée *f* alvéolaire
pyrogenic pyrogène *adj*

Q,R

quarantine quarantenaire *adj*
quinine quinine *f*
rabies; hydrophobia la rage
 ▪ antirabies vaccination = vaccination antirabique
rachitic rachitique *adj*
radioactive radioactif,-ive *adj*
radioactivity radioactivité *f*
radiochemical laboratory laboratoire *m* radiochimique
radiography; x-ray photography radiographie *f*, radio *f*
 ▪ to have a chest/lung x-ray = passer une radio des poumons
 ▪ to have an x-ray taken = passer une radiographie
radiological examination (eg by x-rays) examen *m* radiologique
radiologist radiographe *m*; radiologue *m,f*, radiologiste *m,f*
radiology radiologie *f*
radiotherapist radiothérapeute *m,f*
radiotherapy (eg x-ray treatment) radiothérapie *f*
radius [AM: bone of forearm] radius *m* [AM: os de l'avant-bras]
rale (breathing noises); groan râle *m*
rape viol *m*
rape (to) violer *v*
rare disease; rare illness maladie *f* rare
rash rash *m*; éruption *f*
 ▪ to come out in a rash = avoir une éruption
rash; redness rougeur *f*
Raynaud's disease [AM: vascular spasm of extremities] maladie de Raynaud
 [AM: troubles vasomoteurs des extrémités]
razor rasoir *m*
 ▪ battery shaver = rasoir à piles
 ▪ disposable razor = rasoir jetable
 ▪ electric shaver = rasoir électrique
 ▪ razor; safety razor = rasoir mécanique
 ▪ safety razor = rasoir de sûreté
razor blade lame *f* de rasoir
reaction réaction *f*
 ▪ positive reaction of a skin test = virage d'une cuti-réaction
 ▪ skin test; Heaf test = cuti-réaction *f*
recessive récessif,-ive *adj*
recipient receveur *m*; receveuse *f*
 ▪ universal recipient = receveur universel

recover (to); recuperate (to)   récupérer *v*
recovery (eg from illness)   guérison *f*
recovery: recuperation   récupération *f*
rectitis   rectite *f*
rectoscope   rectoscope *m*
rectoscopy   rectoscopie *f*
rectum; back passage   rectum *m*
recuperate from (to)   se rétablir *v* de
recur (to)   récidiver *v*
recurrence   récidive *f*
recurrent   récurrent,-e *adj*
recurring   récidivant,-e *adj*
recurring (eg fever); periodic   périodique *adj*
recurring nature   récidivité *f*
red blood cell   hématie *f*, érythrocyte *m*; globule *m* rouge
red spots   taches *fpl* rouges
redness; red blotch; red patch   rougeur *f*
reductible   réductible *adj*
reduction; setting (eg of a fracture)   réduction *f*
reflexology   réflexologie *f*
regression   régression *f*
regurgitation   régurgitation *f*
rehabilitate (to); re-educate (to)   rééduquer *v*
rehabilitate (to); readjust (to)   réadapter *v*
rehabilitation; physiotherapy   rééducation *f*
   ▪ speech therapy = rééducation de la parole
   ▪ to undergo/have physiotherapy = faire de la rééducation
reimbursement; refund   remboursement *m*
rejection (eg of graft); vomiting   rejet *m*
relapse   rechute *f*
   ▪ to have a relapse = faire/avoir une rechute
relapse (to); have a relapse (to)   rechuter *v*
relaxant; relaxing   relaxant *m*; relaxant,-e *adj*
relaxation   relaxation *f*; détente *f*
   ▪ a half-hour of relaxation = une demi-heure de détente
remedy, cure; medicine   remède *m*
remission (eg of illness); subsidence; lowering (eg of fever); abatement (eg of pain)   rémission *f*
removal (eg of an organ)   ablation *f*, enlèvement *m*
removal of unwanted hair; epilation   épilation *f*
   ▪ waxing = épilation à la cire

182

remove (to); take out (to) (eg organ) enlever *v;* faire *v* l'ablation de
remove unwanted hair (to) épiler *v*
removing plaster déplâtrage *m*
- taking a limb out of plaster/its plaster cast = le déplâtrage d'un membre
renal rénal,-e *adj*
- acute renal failure = insuffisance rénale aiguë
- renal dialysis = dialyse *f* rénale
- renal failure = défaillance rénale; insuffisance rénale
reopen (to); revive (to) (eg pain,grief) raviver *v*
rescue sauvetage *m*
- life-saving training = cours de sauvetage
resolve (to) (eg tumour) résoudre *v*
resorb (to) résorber *v*
respiration frequency; breathing rate fréquence *f* respiratoire
respirator respirateur *m*
respirator mask masque *m* respiratoire
respiratory respiratoire *adj*
- respiratory affection = affection respiratoire
- respiratory distress syndrome; respiratory difficulties = détresse *f* respiratoire
- respiratory failure = arrêt *m* respiratoire
- respiratory system; respiratory tract = système respiratoire; appareil respiratoire
rest (to) se reposer *v*
resuscitate (to) réanimer *v*
resuscitation réanimation *f*
resuscitator; respirator réanimateur *m*
retention (eg of urine) rétention *f*
retina (eye) rétine *f*
- to become detached (retina) = se décoller *v*
retinitis rétinite *f*
retractor écarteur *m*
retrovirus rétrovirus *m*
revulsion révulsion *f*
Rhesus Rhésus *m*
- Rhesus incompatibility (of blood) = incompatibilité *f* Rhésus
- Rhesus or Rh factor = facteur Rhésus
- Rhesus (Rh) positive/negative = Rhésus positif/négatif
rheumatic rhumatismal,-e *adj*
rheumatism rhumatisme *m*
- acute articular rheumatism = rhumatisme *m* articulaire aigu
- muscular rheumatism = myodynie *f*

183

- rheumatism in the joints; articular rheumatism = rhumatisme *m* articulaire
- rheumatoid arthritis = rhumatisme *m* chronique polyarticulaire

rheumatoid   rhumatoïde *adj*
rheumatoid arthritis   polyarthrite *f* chronique évolutive; PCE; polyarthrite *f* rhumatoïde
rheumatologist   rhumatologiste *m,f*; rhumatologue *m,f*
rheumatology   rhumatologie *f*
rhinitis   [AM: inflammation of the nose]   rhinite *f* (syn. coryza)   [AM: inflammation des fosses nasales]
rhinopharyngitis   rhinopharyngite *f*
rib   côte *f*
riboflavin   riboflavine *f*
ribonucleic acid   acide *m* ribonucléique
rickets; rachitis   rachitisme *m*
- to have rickets; to suffer from rickets = être rachitique

rickettsiosis   rickettsiose *f*
rigor mortis   rigidité *f* cadavérique
ring (under the eye)   cerne *m* (autour des yeux)
ringing (in ears); buzzing   bourdonnement *m*
- ringing in the ears = bourdonnement d'oreilles

ringworm; tinea   teigne *f*
roof of the mouth; bony palate   voûte *f* palatine; voûte *f* du palais
root   racine *f*
- root (of a tooth) = racine dentaire/d'une dent

rosacea   rosacée *f*
roseola (eruption)   roséole *f*
roundworm   ascaride *m*
royal jelly   gelée *f* royale
rubella; German measles   rubéole *f*
rupture   rupture *f*
- rupture of a tendon; tearing of a tendon = rupture tendineuse

rusk   biscuit *m* pour bébés

S

saccharin   sacharine *f*
sacrum   sacrum *m*
safety glasses   lunettes *fpl* de sécurité

safety goggles lunettes *fpl* de protection
safety helmet; hard hat casque *m* de sécurité
safety pin épingle *f* de sûreté
saliva salive *f*
salivary glands glandes *fpl* salivaires
salmonella [AM: bacteria] salmonella *f*, salmonelle *f* [AM: bactéries]
salmonellosis [AM: infection due to salmonella] salmonellose *f* [AM: infection causée par les salmonelles]
salpingitis [AM: inflammation of 1 Fallopian tube; 2 Eustachian tube] salpingite *f* [AM: inflammation de 1 la trompe de Fallope; 2 la trompe d'Eustache]
sample; sampling prélèvement *m*
  ■ I would like a specimen of your blood/ stools/ urine = je voudrais un prélèvement de votre sang/de vos selles/de votre urine
  ■ to take a blood sample = faire un prélèvement de sang
sanatorium maison *f* de cure; sanatorium *m*
sanitary towel serviette *f* hygiénique; serviette périodique
sarcoidosis sarcoïdose *f*
sarcoma [AM: malignant tumour] sarcome *m* [AM: tumeur maligne]
sauna sauna *m*
scab croûte *f*
scabies; itch gale *f*
scald (to) ébouillanter *v*
  ■ to scald oneself = s'ébouillanter
  ■ to scald one's hand = s'ébouillanter la main
scale; squama squame *f*
scalp cuir *m* chevelu
scalpel scalpel *m*
scan scanneur *m*
  ■ to have a scan = passer un scanneur
scan (to) (ultrasonically) échographier *v*
scanner scanneur *m*; scanographe *m*; scanner *m*
scanning; scan scanographie *f*
  ■ to have a scan = passer une scanographie
scapula;scapular (adj) scapulaire *m*; also *adj*
scar cicatrice *f*
  ■ scar tissue = tissus *mpl* cicatrisés
scarificator scarificateur *m*
scarify (to) scarifier *v*
scarlet fever; scarlatina scarlatine *f*
Scheuermann's disease [AM: degenerative affection of vertebral column] maladie de Scheuermann [AM: affection dégénérative de la colonne vertébral]

schizophrenia schizophrénie *f*
schizophrenic schizophrène *adj*
sciatic nerve nerf *m* sciatique
sciatica; sciatic *(adj)* sciatique *f*; also *adj*
scintigraphy scintigraphie *f*
scissors ciseaux *mpl*
sclera; sclerotic [AM: outer membrane of eye] sclérotique *f* (syn. sclère *f*) [AM: membrane qui enveloppe l'œil]
scleroderma sclérodermie *f*
sclerosis sclérose *f*
- hardening of the arteries; arteriosclerosis = sclérose artérielle
- multiple sclerosis = sclérose multiple
- multiple sclerosis; disseminated sclerosis = sclérose en plaques
sclerotic, to become scléroser (se) *v*
scotch test scotch-test *m*
scrape (to) cureter *v*; racler *v*
screening dépistage *m*
- early detection; early screening = dépistage précoce
- mass screening for Aids = dépistage systématique pour sida
scrofula scrofule *f*
scrotal scrotal,-e *adj*
scrotum scrotum *m*; bourses *fpl*
scrub (cosmet) gommage *m*
- to have a body/facial scrub = se faire faire un gommage du corps/du visage
scurf; dead skin peau *f* morte
scurvy; scorbutus scorbut *m*
sea sickness mal *m* de mer
sebaceous cyst kyste *m* sébacé; loupe *f*
sebaceous gland glande *f* sébacée
seborrhoea séborrhée *f*
sebum sébum *m*
secretion sécrétion *f*
sedation sédation *f*
sedative sédatif *m*; sédatif,-ive *adj*
sediment sédiment *m*
seep (to); ooze (out) (to) (eg pus) écouler *v*
seepage infiltration *f*
seizure; attack accès *m*
- attack/bout of fever = accès de fièvre
- attack of coughing = accès de toux
semen sperme *m*; semence *f*

semen analysis spermogramme *m*
senile sénile *adj*
senility sénilité *f*
sensation sensation *f*
sense sens *m*
sensitive sensitif,-ive *adj*
sensitivity sensibilité *f*, réceptivité *f*
 ▪ sensitivity to = réceptivité à
sensitization; sensitizing sensibilisation *f*
sensitized sensibilisé,-e *adj*
sepsis septicité *f*, état *m* septique
septicaemia; septicemia; blood poisoning septicémie *f*
septum (of nose) cloison *f* (du nez)
serenity sérénité *f*
serious grave *adj*; sérieux,-ieuse *adj*
serous séreux,-euse *adj*
serous membrane membrane *f* séreuse
serum sérum *m*
 ▪ antidiphtheria serum = sérum antidiphtérique
 ▪ antitetanus serum = sérum antitétanique
 ▪ blood serum = sérum sanguin
 ▪ physiological solution = sérum physiologique
 ▪ snakebite serum = sérum antivenimeux
set (to) (a fracture) consolider *v* (une fracture)
set (to); reduce (to) (eg fracture) réduire *v*
seton [AM: cotton fibre drainage plug in a wound] séton *m* (à méche) [AM: mèche en coton servant de drain une plaie]
severely ill patient grand malade *m*
sew up (to); stitch (to); suture (to) suturer *v*
sex sexe *m*
sex therapist sexologue *m,f*
sexology sexologie *f*
sexual sexuel,-elle *adj*; sexué,-e *adj*
sexuality sexualité *f*
shadow on the lung voile *m* au poumon
shake (to); shock (to) choquer *v*
 ▪ to be in shock = être choqué
shampoo shampooing *m*
 ▪ shampoo gel = gel shampooing
shave (to) raser *v*
shaving brush blaireau *m*

187

shaving cream   crème *f* à raser
shaving foam   mousse *f* à raser
shinbone   tibia *m*
shingles; herpes zoster   zona *m*; herpés *m* zoster
shiver (to) (eg with fever)   frissonner *v*
shiver (with) (to) (eg cold, fever)   grelotter *v* (de); trembler *v*
shock   choc *m*
  ▪ anaphylactic shock = choc anaphylactique
  ▪ cardiac shock = choc cardiogénique
  ▪ electric shock = choc électrique
  ▪ in a state of shock = en état de choc
  ▪ (nervous) shock = choc nerveux
  ▪ post-operative shock = choc opératoire
  ▪ she is suffering from shock = elle est sous le coup de choc
shock   commotion *f*
  ▪ electric shock = commotion électrique
  ▪ mental shock = commotion mentale
shooting pain; sharp pain; twinge   élancement *m*
shoulder   épaule *f*
  ▪ frozen shoulder = épaule bloquée
shoulder blade   omoplate *f*; scapulaire *m*; also *adj*
shunt   shunt *m*
sibilant (whistling)   sibilant,-e *adj*
sick leave   congé *m* de maladie
sick; ill   malade *adj*
  ▪ seriously/critically ill = gravement malade
  ▪ to be ill/sick = être malade
sickness   maladie *f*; mal *m*; vomissements *mpl* (nausea)
side effects   effets *mpl* secondaires
sight test   test *m* d'acuité visuelle
sight testing chart   tableau *m* d'acuité visuelle
sigmoid colon   sigmoïde *m*; also *adj*
silicone   silicone *f*
silicosis   silicose *f*
sinus   sinus *m*
sinusitis   sinusite *f*
siphon   siphon *m*
sizzling; crackling (noise)   grésillement *m*
skeleton   squelette *m*
skin   peau *f*
  ▪ greasy/dry skin = peau grasse/sèche

- skin bank = banque *f* de peau
- skin complaint/disease = maladie *f* de peau
- skin peeling treatment = peeling *m*
- slack/loose skin = peau relâchée

skull crâne *m*; boîte *f* crânienne

sleep sommeil *m*

sleep inducing hypnotique *m*; also *adj*

sleeping pill somnifère *m*

sleepwalk (to) marcher *v* en dormant; être *v* somnambule

sleepwalker somnambule *m,f*
- she sleepwalks = elle est somnambule

sleepwalking somnambulisme *m*

slim (to) maigrir *v*
- she is on a slimming programme = elle suit un régime pour maigrir
- to be on a slimming diet = suivre un régime amaigrissant

slim; slender mince *adj*

slimmer (to get) amincir (s') *v*

slimming amincissement *m*

slimming amincissant,-e *adj*
- slimming product = produit amincissant

slimness; slenderness minceur *f*

sling (bandage) écharpe *f*
- in a sling = en écharpe

slipped disc hernie *f* discale

small pox vaccine vaccin *m* antivariolique

smallpox variole *f*

smear frottis *m*
- blood smear = frottis sanguin
- to have a cervical smear = se faire faire un frottis cervicovaginal

smell, sense of odorat *m*
- he has a keen sense of smell = il a l'odorat fin

smooth; creamy onctueux,-euse *adj*

sneeze (to) éternuer *v*

sneeze; sneezing éternuement *m*

snore (to) ronfler *v*

snoring ronflement *m*; ronflements *mpl*

soap savon *m*
- baby's soap = savon pour bébés
- dermatological soap = savon dermatologique
- household soap = savon de Marseille
- liquid soap = savon liquide

- mild soap = savon doux
- scented soap = savon parfumé
- shaving soap = savon à barbe
- soft soap = savon mou
- toilet soap = savon de toilette

socket (of bone)   cavité *f* articulaire
sodium bicarbonate   bicarbonate *m* de sodium
soften   ramoir *v*
softening   ramollissement *m*
sole (of the foot)   plante *f* (du pied)
solution   solution *f*
soothing   apaisant,-e *adj*
- soothing cream/lotion/powder = crème/lotion/poudre apaisante

soporific   somnifère *m*
soporific   soporifique *adj*
sore throat   mal *m* à la gorge
sore; wound   plaie *f*
spa   station *f* thermale
Spanish flu   grippe *f* espagnole
spasm   spasme *m*
- clonic spasm = spasme clonique
- epileptic spasm (baby) = spasme en flexion
- tonic spasm = spasme tonique

spatula   spatule *f*
specialist   spécialiste *m,f*
speculum   spéculum *m*
speech therapy   orthophonie *f*
sperm; semen   sperme *m*; semence *f*
sperm bank   banque *f* de sperme
spermicide   spermicide *m*; also *adj*
sphincter   sphincter *m*
sphygmomanometer   [AM: instrument for measuring blood pressure]   sphygmo-manomètre *m*; tensiomètre *m*   [AM: appareil servant à mesurer la pression artérielle]
spina bifida   spina-bifida *m*
spinal bulb   bulbe *m* rachidien
spinal chord; spinal marrow   moelle *f* épinière; corde *f* spinale
spinal column   colonne vertébrale *f*
spinal meningitis   méningite *f* cérébro-spinale
spinal nerve   nerf *m* rachidien
spine   colonne *f* vertébrale
spleen   rate *f*

splint attelle *f*; éclisse *f*; gouttière *f*
- sagittal suture = gouttière sagittale
- vertebral groove = gouttière vertébrale

splinter écharde *f*

splinting; fixing bones with screwed plates éclissage *m*

splints, to put in éclisser *v*

spondylitis [AM: inflammation of a vertebra] spondylite *f* [AM: inflammation d'une vertèbre]

spondylopathy [AM: all disease of the spinal column] spondylopathie *f* [AM: toute affection de la colonne vertébrale]

sponge éponge *f*

spore (eg fungus, bacterium) spore *f*

spot; pimple bouton *m*

sprain entorse *f*; foulure *f*
- to sprain one's wrist = se faire une entorse au poignet

sprain (to); twist (to) fouler (se) *v*
- to have a sprained ankle = avoir la cheville foulé
- to twist or sprain one's wrist/ankle = se fouler le poignet/la cheville

spray bombe *f* (aérosol)
- can (aerosol) of shaving cream = bombe à raser

spray spray *m*

spray; atomizer vaporisateur *m*; vapo *m*
- perfume spray/atomizer = vaporisateur à parfum

spreading (eg pain) rayonnant,-e *adj*

sprue sprue *f*

squamous; squamose squameux,-euse *adj*

stagefright; (exam) nerves trac *m*

stammering; stuttering bégaiment *m*

staphylococcia staphylococcie *f*

staphylococcus (bacterium) staphylocoque *m*
- staphylococcus aureus = staphylocoque doré

stenosis sténose *f*; rétrécissement *m*

steppage gait steppage *m*

sterile stérile *adj*

sterile compress tricostéril *m*

sterility stérilité *f*

sterilization stérilisation *f*

sterilize (to) stériliser *v*

sterilize (to) (in a flame) flamber *v*

sterilizer stérilisateur *m*

sterilizing solution solution *f* de stérilisation

sternum; breast bone sternum *m*

steroid stéroïde *m*; also *adj*
- steroidal hormone = stéroïde hormonal

stethoscope stéthoscope *m*

stick (cosmet) stick *m*
- shaving stick = stick à raser

stiff neck torticolis *m*

stigma; mark; scar stigmate *m*

stillbirth enfant *m* mort-né; enfant *f* mort-née

sting; bite (of insect) piqûre *f*
- bee/wasp sting = piqûre d'abeille/de guêpe
- insect bite = piqûre d'insecte
- jellyfish sting = piqûre de méduse

sting (to) (insect) piquer *v*

stirrup étrier *m*

stitch (to); sew up (to) suturer *v*; recoudre *v*

stitch [AM: pain in the side] point *m* de côté [AM: douleur localisée sur le côté]
- avoir le point de côté = to have the stitch

stitch up again (to); put stitches back in (to) (eg wound) recoudre *v*

stomach estomac *m*; ventre *m*
- distension of the stomach = gonflement du ventre
- I have an upset stomach = j'ai mal au ventre
- I have a pain in my stomach = j'ai mal au ventre
- stomach ache = mal *m* à l'estomac; mal d'estomac

stomach muscles abdominaux *mpl*
- to exercise the stomach muscles = faire des abdominaux

stomach pump pompe *f* stomacale

stomach, on an empty jeun; à jeun *adv*
- to be taken on an empty stomach = à prendre à jeun

stomatitis stomatite *f*

stomatologist stomatologiste *m,f*; stomatologue *m,f*

stomatology [AM: study of diseases of the mouth and teeth] stomatologie *f* [AM: étude des maladies de la bouche et des dents]

stomy stomie *f*

stone pierre *f*

stools; motions selles *fpl*
- have you had or passed a motion today? = êtes-vous allé à la selle aujourd'hui?

strabismus [AM: eyesight defect] strabisme *m* [AM: défaut de la vision]

strain (muscular) froissement *m* (d'un muscle)

strain (to) (eg a muscle) froisser (se) *v*

strawberry; strawberry mark fraise *f*

streptococcia [AM: infection by streptococci bacteria] streptococcie *f* [AM: infection due aux streptocoques]

streptococcus (bacterium) streptocoque *m*
streptomycin streptomycine *f*
stress stress *m, inv*
stress, to put under stresser *v*
stressful stressant,-e *adj*
stretch marks vergetures *fpl*
stretcher civière *f*, brancard *m*
stretching (eg of muscle); extension; traction (eg of limb) extension *f*
stricture (eg of intestine) rétrécissement *m*
stroke ; cerebrovascular accident accident *m* vasculaire cérébral; infarctus
   cérébral; ramollissement *m* cérébral
stupefy (to) stupéfier *v*
stupefying stupéfiant,-e *adj*
stupor stupeur *f*
sty(e) compère-loriot; orgelet *m*
stylet; stilette (small probe) stylet *m*
subsidence; lowering (eg of fever) rémission *f*
suction; sucking succion *f*
sudden; violent brutal,-e *adj*
   ▪ a sudden obstruction of a coronary artery = une obstruction brutale d'une artère
   coronaire
suffer (to) souffrir *v*
suffocation étouffement *m*; suffocation *f*
   ▪ he had fits of choking = il avait des suffocations
   ▪ to die of suffocation = mourir d'étouffement
sulphonamide; sulfonamide sulfamide *m*
sun soleil *m*; solaire *adj*
   ▪ sun block = crème écran total
   ▪ sunburn; slight sunstroke = coup de soleil
   ▪ sunscreen = écran *m* solaire
   ▪ suntan cream = crème *f* solaire
   ▪ suntan lotion factor 8 = crème solaire facteur 8
   ▪ suntan lotion = lotion *f* solaire
   ▪ suntan oil = huile *f* solaire
sun-tanning; tan bronzage *m*
sunglasses lunettes *fpl* de soleil
sunstroke insolation *f*
   ▪ she has got sunstroke = elle a une insolation
   ▪ to get sunstroke = attraper une insolation
support (eg bandage, splint, plaster, brace) contention *f*
suppository suppositoire *m*

193

suppurate suppurer *v*

suppuration [AM: formation of pus] suppuration *f* [AM: formation de pus]

surgeon chirurgien *m*, chirurgienne *f*

surgery (place) cabinet *m* médical

surgery (action) chirurgie *f*

surgical chirurgical,-e *adj*

surgical corset ceinture *f* orthopédique

surgical masque masque *m* de gaze

surgical removal (of an organ) ablation *f* chirurgicale

surgical spirit alcool *m* à 90 (degrés); alcool modifié à 90

surrogate mother mère *f* porteuse

suture suture *f*

suture (to) suturer *v*

swab (medical) tampon *m*

swallow (to) avaler *v*; déglutir *v*
  ▪ not to be taken internally = ne pas avaler

swallowing act of, deglutition déglutition *f*

sweat gland glande *f* sudoripare

sweetener, artificial édulcorant *m* de synthèse

swell up (to); become puffy (to) (face, eyelid) gonfler *v*; enfler *v*

swell up again (to) regonfler *v*

swelling enflure *f*

swelling (eg eyelid, feet); distension (eg stomach) gonflement *m*

swelling; inflammation; congestion fluxion *f*
  ▪ pneumonia = fluxion de poitrine
  ▪ swelling; gumboil = fluxion dentaire

swimming natation *f*

sycosis [AM: infection of the beard area] sycosis *m* [AM: infection à la zone de la barbe]

symptom symptôme *m*

symptomatic symptomatique *adj*

synapse synapse *f*

syndrome syndrome *m*
  ▪ acquired immunodeficiency syndrome = syndrome immunodéficitaire acquis
  ▪ Down's syndrome = syndrome de Down
  ▪ Toxic Shock Syndrome = syndrome du choc toxique; SCT

synergistic synergiste *m*; also *adj*

synergy synergie *f*

synovia synovie *f*
  ▪ to have water on the knee = avoir un épanchement de synovie

synovial synovial,-ale *adj*
  ▪ synovial fluid; synovial liquid = liquide *m* synovial

194

synovial membrane synoviale *f*
syphilis syphilis *f*
syringe seringue *f*
system système *m*
systemic systémique *adj*
systemic acute lupus erythematosis lupus *m* érythémateux aigu disséminé

T

tablet cachet *m*
- aspirin tablet = cachet d'aspirine
- chewable tablet = cachet à croquer
- soluble tablet = cachet soluble
- take two tablets a day after meals = prenez deux cachets par jour après les repas

tablet comprimé *m*
- coated tablet = comprimé pelliculé
- take the tablets before/after meals = prenez les comprimés avant/après les repas
- take the tablets in the morning/at night = prenez les comprimés le matin/le soir
- take the tablets with water = prenez les comprimés avec un verre d'eau
- under-tongue tablet = comprimé sublingual (= linguette)

tachycardia [AM: greatly raised pulse rate] tachycardie *f* [AM: acceleration du rythme cardiaque]

take (to) (eg sample) prélever *v*
- to remove an organ = prélever un organe
- to remove from = prélever sur
- to take a sample of (eg blood) = prélever un échantillon de

take (to); catch (to) (eg a cold) prendre *v*
- to be taken before meals = à prendre avant les repas
- to be taken three times a day = à prendre matin, midi et soir
- to be taken three times a day = à prendre trois fois par jour
- to catch a cold = prendre un rhume

take out of plaster (to) déplâtrer *v*

taken pris, prise *adj*
- my nose is stuffed up = j'ai le nez pris
- my throat is hoarse = j'ai la gorge prise

talc; talcum powder talc *m*

tamponade; tamponage tamponnement *m*

tampon tampon *m* hygiénique

tapeworm; taenia [AM: parasitic worm] ténia *m*; taenia *m*; ver *m* solitaire [AM: ver parasite]

195

tapotement; tapping or percussion massage tapotement *m*
- to tap = tapoter *v*

tarsus tarse *m*
- tarsals = os du tarse

tartar tartre *m*

taste goût *m*

taste buds; lingual papillae papilles *fpl* linguales; papilles *fpl* gustatives

tattoo; tattooing tatouage *m*

tear (to) (eg a muscle) déchirer (se) *v*
- to tear a muscle = se déchirer un muscle

tear ducts voies *fpl* lacrymales

tear; laceration déchirure *f*
- abdominal/intercostal/ muscle tear = déchirure abdominale/intercostale/ musculaire

teaspoonful (eg of medicine) cuillerée *f* à café
- take two teaspoonfuls after meals = prenez deux cuillerées après les repas
- tablespoonful = cuillerée à soupe

teat (of baby's bottle) tétine *f*

teeth; dentition; teething dentition *f*

teething ring anneau *m* de dentition

tegument tégument *m*

teleradiotherapy téléradiothérapie *f*

temperature température *f*
- to have a temperature = avoir/faire de la température
- to take someone's temperature = prendre la température de quelqu'un

temperature chart feuille *f* de température

temple tempe *f*

tendon; sinew (muscle tendon) tendon *m*

tennis elbow; epicondylitis épicondylite *f*

tent (surgery); wick; pack mèche *f*
- to tent a wound = introduire une meche dans une plaie

term terme *m*
- full-term delivery = accouchement à terme
- to be born/delivered prematurely = naître/accoucher avant terme

tertiary tertiaire *adj*

test test *m*

test; trial épreuve *f*

testicle testicule *m*
- torsion of the testicle = torsion du testicule

testosterone [AM: male hormone] testostérone *f* [AM: hormone stéroïde mâle]

tetanus tétanos *m*

■ have you been inoculated against tetanus? = êtes-vous vacciné(e) contre le tétanos?

tetany tétanie *f*

tetracycline [AM: antibiotic} tétracycline *f* [AM: antibiotique]

thalamus [AM: part of brain] thalamus *m* [AM: partie du cerveau]

thalassotherapy; marine therapy thalassothérapie *f*; thérapie *f* marine

therapeutics; treatment; therapeutic *(adj)* thérapeutique *f*; also *adj*

therapy thérapie *f*

thermometer thermomètre *m*
■ Celsius/centigrade /Fahrenheit thermometer = thermomètre Celsius/centigrade/Fahrenheit
■ thermometer, clinical = thermomètre *m* médical

thermotherapy; heat treatment thermothérapie *f*
■ to treat by thermotherapy = traiter par la thermothérapie

thigh cuisse *f*

thin maigre *adj*

third finger annulaire *m*

thirst soif *f*

thoracic cage; rib cage cage *f* thoracique

thoracic duct canal *m* thoracique

thorax thorax *m*

thready (eg pulse) filiforme *adj*

throat gorge *f*
■ I have a sore throat = j'ai mal à la gorge

throat infection; tonsillitis; pharyngitis; angina angine *f*
■ to have a sore throat = avoir une angine

throat pastilles pastilles *fpl* pour la gorge

thrombin thrombine *f*

thrombosis thrombose *f*

thrush; white mouth muguet *m* (buccal)

thrush (vaginal) mycose *f* vaginale; mycose à candida albicans; muguet *m* vaginal

thumb pouce *m*

thymic thymique *adj*

thymus [AM: gland involved in lymphocytes production] thymus *m* [AM: glande dont la fonction est de produire des lymphocytes]

thyroid; thyroid gland thyroïde *f* also *adj*; glande *f* thyroïde

tibia tibia *m*

tic tic *m*

tincture teinture *f*
■ alcoholic tincture = teinture alcoolique

197

toothpaste

- tincture of iodine = teinture d'iode
tinnitus aurium (ear) acouphène *m*
tinting/colouring product for hair produit *m* de coloration
tissue tissu *m*
- connective tissue = tissu conjonctif
tissues; paper hankerchiefs mouchoirs *mpl* en papier
tobacco addiction; nicotine poisoning (intoxication); tabagism tabagisme *m*; nicotinisme *m*
toe orteil *m*; doigt *m* de pied
- big toe = gros orteil
toenail ongle *m* de l'orteil; ongle *m* du pied
toilet paper papier *m* hygiénique; papier *m* toilette
tolerance tolérance *f*
tolerate (to) tolérer *v*
tomography [AM: radiological method for sectional scanning of body] tomographie *f* [AM: methode radiologique permettant la visualisation des structures anatomique]
tone; tonicity; tonus tonicité *f*
tongue langue *f*
- open your mouth; put your tongue out = ouvrez la bouche; tirez la langue
- to have a coated or furred tongue = avoir la langue blanche/chargée
tonic tonique *m*; also *adj*
tonic; antidepressant remontant *m*
tonsil tonsille *f*
tonsillectomy [AM: tonsil removal] amygdalectomie *f*; tonsillectomie *f* [AM: ablation des amygdales]
tonsillitis amygdalite *f*; tonsillite *f*
tonsils amygdales *fpl*
tooth, teeth *(pl)* dent *f*; dents *fpl*
- hollow tooth = dent creuse
- milk tooth; baby tooth = dent de lait
- set of teeth = denture *f*
- to brush one's teeth = se brosser les dents
- to fill a tooth temporarily = panser une dent
- wisdom tooth = dent de sagesse
tooth extraction avulsion *f* dentaire
tooth powder poudre *f* dentifrice
toothache mal *m* de dents; rage *f* de dents
- I have a toothache = j'ai mal aux dents
toothbrush brosse *f* à dents
toothpaste; dentifrice dentifrice *m*; also *adj*; pâte *f* dentifrice
- fluoride toothpaste = dentifrice fluoré
- tooth powder = poudre dentifrice

toothpick cure-dents *m*
topical; local topique *adj*
torsion; twisting torsion *f*
torticollis; wry neck torticolis *m*
touch, sense of toucher *m*
  ▪ rectal/vaginal examination (using fingers) = un toucher rectal/vaginal
tourniquet garrot *m*; tourniquet *m*
toxaemia; toxemia toxémie *f*
toxic toxique *adj*
toxicologist toxicologue *m,f*
toxicology toxicologie *f*
toxin toxine *f*
toxoplasmosis toxoplasmose *f*
tracer marqueur *m*
trachea trachée *f*
tracheotomy trachéotomie *f*
trachoma [AM: eye infection] trachome *m* [AM: infection de l'œil]
tract (eg digestive) appareil *m*; voie *f*
traction traction *f*; élongation *f*; extension *f*
  ▪ in traction = en traction
traffic accident service service *m* de secours aux victimes de la circulation
tranquillizer calmant *m*; tranquillisant *m*
tranquillizer; tranquillizing tranquillisant,-e *adj*
transfuse (to) transfuser *v*
transfusion transfusion *f*
transmit (to); pass on (to) (eg disease) transmettre *v*
transplant (to) transplanter *v*
transplant (to); graft (to) greffer *v*
transplant; graft greffe *f*
  ▪ kidney transplant = greffe de rein
  ▪ organ transplant = greffe d'organes
  ▪ skin graft = greffe de peau
transplantation; transplant transplantation *f*
  ▪ heart/kidney transplant = transplantation cardiaque/du rein
trauma trauma *m*
traumatic traumatique *adj*
traumatism traumatisme *m*
travel sickness; motion sickness mal *m* des transports
  ▪ travel-sickness pill = comprimé *m* contre le mal des transports
treat (to) (eg an illness) traiter *v*; soigner *v*
treatment traitement *m*

typhus

- to be having treatment (ie in hospital) = être en traitement
treatment; care; after-treatment   soins *mpl*
  - cleansing treatments = soins nettoyants
  - hair care = soins du cheveux
  - intensive care = soins intensifs
  - skin care; facial care = soins du visage
  - statement of treatment = feuille *f* de soins
  - to be under treatment = être en traitement
tremor   trémor *m*; tremblement *m*; trémulation *f*
trepan (to); trephine (to)   trépaner *v*
trepan; trephine   trépan *m*
trepanation; trephination   trépanation *f*
triceps (muscles)   triceps *m*
tropical disease   maladie *f* tropicale
trouble; disorder   trouble *m*
  - digestive disorders = troubles digestifs
  - physiological disorders = troubles physiologiques
  - sleep disorders = troubles du sommeil
  - speech difficulties = troubles du langage
trance; catalepsy   catalepsie *f*
  - to fall or go into a trance = tomber en catalepsie
trunk   tronc *m*
truss   bandage *m* herniaire; ceinture *f* herniaire
tubal   tubaire *adj*
tubercle   tubercule *m*
tuberculosis   tuberculose *f*
tuberculous; tubercular   tuberculeux,-euse *adj*
  - to suffer from tuberculosis = être tuberculeux
tumour   tumeur *f*
tweezers   pince *f* à échardes
tweezers (eyebrow)   pince *f* à épiler
twins; twin (male, female)   jumeaux *mpl*; jumeau *m*; jumelle *f*
typhoid; typhoid fever   typhoïde *f*, fièvre *f* typhoïde
typhus   typhus *m*

U

ulcer ulcère *m*
- to have a stomach ulcer = avoir un ulcère à l'estomac

ulcerate (to) ulcérer *v*
- ulcerated wound = plaie ulcérée
- wound that ulcerates or festers = blessure qui s'ulcère

ulceration ulcération *f*

ulcerous; covered in ulcers ulcéreux,-euse *adj*

ulna [AM: inner bone of forearm] cubitus *m* [AM: os interne de l'avant-bras]

ultrasonic échographique *adj*; ultrasonique *adj*

ultrasound ultrason *m*

ultrasound cardiography échocardiographie *m*

ultrasound scan échographie *f*
- to have an ultrasonic scan = passer une échographie
- to have an ultrasound scan = se faire faire une échographie

ultrasound scanner échographe *m*

ultraviolet ultraviolet,-ette *adj*
- to receive ultraviolet treatment = se faire traiter aux rayons ultraviolets
- ultraviolet radiation = rayonnement ultraviolet; rayons *mpl* ultraviolets

unbandage (to) débander *v*

unblock (to) (eg intestine) libérer *v*

uncinariasis; hookworm disease ankylostomiase *f*, ankylostomose *f*

unconscious sans connaissance *adj*; évanoui *adj*
- he is unconscious = il s'est évanoui
- he remained unconscious for an hour = il est resté sans connaissance pendant une heure
- to become unconscious = perdre connaissance

unconsciousness perte *f* de connaissance

underarm crutch béquille *f* commune

underweight. maigre *adj*

uneven (pulse) ondulant,-e *adj*

unwell souffrant,-e *adj*
- to be unwell = être souffrant

upper teeth dents *fpl* du haut

upset embarras *m*
- upset stomach; stomach upset = embarras gastrique

urea urée *f*

ureter uretère *m*

urethra urètre *m*

urethritis urétrite *f*

valve

uric acid   acide *m* urique
urinary tract   voies *fpl* urinaires
urine   urine *f*
urine analysis   analyse *f* d'urine
urogenital   urogénital *adj*
urologist   urologue *m,f*
urology   urologie *f*
urticaria; nettlerash; hives   urticaire *f*
use; usage   usage *m*
▪ for external/internal use = à usage externe/interne
uterine contractions   contractions *fpl* utérines
uterography   hystérographie *f*
uterus; womb   utérus *m*; matrice *f*
▪ prolapse of the uterus = descente *f* de l'utérus; descente *f* de matrice
uveal tract (eye)   tractus *m* uvéal; uvée *f*
uvula   luette *f*

V

vaccinate (to); inoculate (to)   vacciner *v*
▪ have you been inoculated against tetanus? = êtes-vous vacciné(e) contre le tétanos?
▪ to have a vaccination = se faire vacciner
vaccination   vaccination *f*
vaccination certificate   certificat *m* de vaccination
vaccination record   carnet *m* de vaccination
vaccine   vaccin *m*
▪ rubella vaccine = vaccin contre la rubéole
▪ yellow fever vaccine = vaccin contre la fièvre jaune
vagal   [AM: relating to vagus nerve]   vagal,-e *adj*   [AM: qui se rapporte au nerf vague]
vagina   vagin *m*
vaginal   vaginal,-ale *adj*
▪ I have a vaginal infection = j'ai une infection vaginale
vaginitis   vaginite *f*
valerian   valériane *f*
valium ®   valium ® *m*
valve   valve *f*
▪ heart valve = valve cardiaque

valve; valvula valvule *f*
- heart valves = valvules cardiaques
valvular valvulaire *adj*
varicose vein; varix varice *f*, varices *fpl*
vas deferens canal *m* déférent
vasectomy [AM: removal of part of the vas deferens] vasectomie *f* [AM: résection partielle des canaux déférents]
vaseline ®; petrolatum vaseline ® *f*
vasoconstriction vasoconstriction *f*
vasoconstrictor; vasoconstrictive nerve vasoconstricteur *m*; vasoconstricteur,-trice *adj*
vasodilation vasodilatation *f*
vasodilator vasodilatateur *m*; vasodilatateur,-trice *adj*
vegan végétalien,-ienne *adj*
veganism végétalisme *m*
vegetarian végétarien,-ienne *adj*
vegetarianism végétarisme *m*
vein veine *f*
- coronary vein = veine *f* coronaire
- jugular vein = veine *f* jugulaire
- portal vein = veine *f* porte
- pulmonary vein = veine *f* pulmonaire
- saphenous; superficial leg vein = saphène *f* (veine); also *adj*
vena cava, inferior veine *f* cave inférieure
vena cava, superior veine *f* cave supérieure
venereal vénérien,-ienne *adj*
- venereal diseases; V.D. = maladies vénériennes
venom (eg snake) venin *m*
venous veineux,-euse *adj*
ventilation ventilation *f*
- respiratory ventilation = ventilation respiratoire
ventricle ventricule *m*
- left/right ventricle (of heart) = ventricule *m* gauche/droite
ventricular ventriculaire *adj*
vermifuge (to remove intestinal worms) vermifuge *m*
vertebra (vertebrae pl) vertèbre *f*
- cervical vertebrae = vertèbres cervicales
- dorsal vertebrae = vertèbres dorsales
- lumbar vertebrae = vertèbres lombaires
vertebral vertebral,-e *adj*
vertebral column colonne *f* vertébrale; colonne *f* rachidienne; rachis *m*

vertebrate vertébré *m*
vertiginous vertigineux,-euse *adj*
vertigo vertige *m*
vesicatory vésicatoire *m*; also *adj*
vesicle; blister vésicule *f*
 ▪ genital warts = vésicules génitales
vibrations; vibromassage vibrations *fpl*
 ▪ vibromassage = traitement par vibrations
vignette see French section
Vincent's angina/disease angine *f* de Vincent
virilism virilisation *f*
virology virologie *f*
virology laboratory laboratoire *m* de virologie
virus virus *m*
viscera viscères *mpl*
visceral viscéral,-e *adj*
vision vision *f*
 ▪ double vision = vision *f* double
vitaliser vitaliseur *m*
vitality vitalité *f*
vitamin vitamine *f*
 ▪ vitamin C = vitamine C
 ▪ vitamin tablet/pill = comprimé *m* de vitamine
 ▪ with added vitamins; vitamin enriched = vitaminé
vocal cord corde *f* vocale
volvulus [AM: twisting of intestine causing blockage] volvulus *m* [AM: torsion de l'intestin provoquant un occlusion]
vomit vomi *m*
vomit (to) vomir *v*
vomiting; vomit vomissement *m*
 ▪ I have been vomiting = j'ai eu des vomissements
 ▪ to start to vomit = être pris de vomissements
vulva vulve *f*
vulvitis vulvite *f*

W

waist   taille *f*

walking frame; walker   cadre *m* de marche

walking stick; cane   canne *f*
- (forearm) crutch = canne anglaise
- quadruped stick = canne avec quadripode
- white stick = canne blanche

wall (eg of stomach)   paroi *f*

ward (in hospital)   service *m*; salle *f* d'hôpital; unité *f*
- he is in ward 5 = il est à unité 5
- maternity ward = service de maternité
- pediatrics ward = service de pédiatrie
- which ward? = quel service?

wart; verruca   verrue *f*
- verruca; plantar wart = verrue plantar

wart remover   verrucide *m*

wash out (to) (eg the intestine)   laver *v*

washing; washing out   lavage *m*
- intestinal wash = lavage d'intestin
- stomach wash = lavage gastrique
- to pump someone's stomach out = faire un lavage d'estomac à quelqu'un

water   eau *f*; eaux *fpl*
- her waters have broken = elle a perdu les eaux

water bed   lit *m* d'eau

waterproof   étanche *adj*

wax   cire *f*
- beeswax = cire d'abeilles
- wax applicator = applicateur de cire
- waxing = épilation à la cire

wax bath   bain *m* de paraffine

weak   faible *adj*

weaning   sevrage *m*

weight   poids *m*

wellbeing; welfare   bien-être *m*

wen; sebaceous cyst   loupe *f*; kyste *m* sébacé

wheat germ oil   huile *f* de germe de blé

wheelchair   fauteuil *m* roulant; fauteuil à roulettes (pour malades)

wheezing   wheezing *m*

whistling; hissing   sifflement *m*
- ringing in the ears; tinnitus = sifflement d'oreilles

zygote

whitlow panaris *m*
whooping cough coqueluche *f*
wide-toothed comb démêloir *m*
windpipe; trachea trachée *f*
wipe one's bottom se torcher *v*
wipe, antiseptic tampon *m* aseptique
wipes (cosmet) lingettes *f*
wipes (baby) lingettes *fpl* de bébé
withdrawal (eg giving up alcohol, drugs etc) sevrage *m*
▪ withdrawal symptoms = symptômes de sevrage
working; functioning fonctionnement *m*
wound blessure *f*; plaie *f*
wrinkle ride *f*
wrist poignet *m*
wrist joint articulation *f* du poignet

XYZ

x-ray (to) radiographier *v*
▪ to have an x-ray taken = se faire radiographier
x-ray department service *m* de radiologie; service *m* radiologique
x-ray examination; radiography examen *m* radiographique
x-ray photograph; radiograph radiographie *f*, radio *f*
▪ you will need to have an X-ray taken = il faut vous faire une radio
yaws; pian pian *m*
yoga yoga *m*
zygote zygote *m*

ail *m*	garlic	Allium sativum
algues *fpl*	algae; seaweed	
ananas *m*	pineapple	Ananas comosus
angelique *f*	angelica, wild	Angelica sylvestris
armoise *f*	artemisia	Artemisia vulgaris
arnica *f*	arnica	Arnica montana
artichaut *m*	artichoke, globe	Cynara scolymus
aubépine *f*	hawthorn	Crataegus oxycantha
badiane *f*, anis *m* étoilé	star anise; Chinese anise	Illicium anisatum
basilic *m*	basil	Ocimum basilicum
bigarade *f*	Seville orange; bitter orange	Citrus aurantium
boldo *m*	boldo	Peumus boldus
bouleau *m*	silver birch	Betula pendula
bourdaine *f*	alder buckthorne	Frangula alnus
bourrache *f* officinale	borage	Borago officinalis
bugrane *f*	restharrow	Ononis spinosa
camomille *f* allemande	German camomile	Matricaria chamomilla
cassis *m*	blackcurrant	Ribes nigrum
chiendent *m*	couch grass	Agropyron repens
chrysanthème *m* des prés	oxeye daisy	Chrysanthemum leucanthemum
citron *m*	lemon	Citrus limon
coquelicot *m*	corn poppy	Papaver rhoeas
cyprès *m*	cypress, Italian	Cupressus sempervirens
dent-de-lion *f*	dandelion	Taraxacum officinale
escholtzie *f*	California poppy	Eschscholtzia californica
fenouil *m*	fennel	Anethum foeniculum
fenugrec *m*	fenugreek	Trigonella foenum-graecum
frêne *m*	ash	Fraxinus excelsior
garcinia *m* / guttier *m*	gamboge	Garcinia Cambogia
gentiane *f* jaune	gentian, yellow	Gentiana lutea
ginkgo biloba *m*	gingko biloba	Gingko biloba

ginseng *m*	gingseng	Panax ginseng
genévrier *m*	juniper	Juniperus communis
griffe *f* du diable (harpagophytum)	devil's claw	Harpagophytum procumbens
groseiller *m* rouge	red currant	Ribes rubrum
hamamélis *m*	witch hazel	Hamamelis virginiana
kava-kava *f*	kavakava	Piper methylsticum
konjac *m*	konjak	Amorphophallus konjac
lavande *f*	lavender	Lavandula spica
marron *m* d'Inde	horse chestnut	Aesculus hippocastanum
mélilot *m*	melilot, yellow; sweet clover	Melilotus officinalis
mélisse *f*	balm	Melissa officinalis
menthe *f* poivrée	peppermint	Mentha x piperita
millefeuille *m*	milfoil; yarrow	Achillea millefolium
millepertuis *m*	St. John's Wort	Hypericum perforatum
myrtille *f*	bilberry; whortleberry	Vaccinium Myrtillus
onagre *f*	evening primrose	Oenothera biennis
origan *m*	marjoram	Origanum vulgare
ortie *f* piquante	stinging nettle	Urtica dioca
papaye *f*	papaya	Carica papaya
passiflore *f*	passiflore; passion flower	Passiflora incarnata
pensée *f* sauvage	heartsease; pansy	Viola tricolor
petite pervenche *f*	lesser periwinkle	Vinca minor
plantain *m* majeur	plantain, greater	Plantago major
prêle *f*	horse-tail	Equisetum arvense
raisin d'ours *m*	bearberry	Arctostaphylos uvi-ursi
reine *f* des prés	meadowsweet	Spiraea ulmaria
rhubarbe *f*	rhubarb	Rheum palmatum
réglisse *f*	liquorice	Glycyrrhiza glabra
romarin *m*	rosemary	Rosmarinus officinalis
salsepareille *f*	sarsaparilla	Smilax aspera
sauge *f*	sage, common	Salvia officinalis
saule *m* blanc	white willow	Salix alba
sené *m*	senna	Cassia angustifolia

valériane *f*	valerian	Valeriana officinalis
vergerette *f* de Canada	fleabane, Canadian	Erigeron Canadensis
vigne *f* rouge	vine	Vitis vinifera

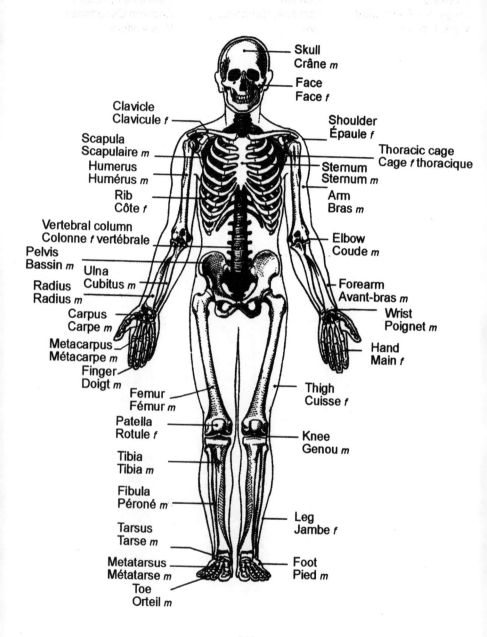

Skull
Crâne *m*

Face
Face *f*

Clavicle
Clavicule *f*

Shoulder
Épaule *f*

Scapula
Scapulaire *m*

Thoracic cage
Cage *f* thoracique

Humerus
Humérus *m*

Sternum
Sternum *m*

Rib
Côte *f*

Arm
Bras *m*

Vertebral column
Colonne *f* vertébrale

Elbow
Coude *m*

Pelvis
Bassin *m*

Ulna
Cubitus *m*

Radius
Radius *m*

Forearm
Avant-bras *m*

Wrist
Poignet *m*

Carpus
Carpe *m*

Metacarpus
Métacarpe *m*

Hand
Main *f*

Finger
Doigt *m*

Femur
Fémur *m*

Thigh
Cuisse *f*

Patella
Rotule *f*

Knee
Genou *m*

Tibia
Tibia *m*

Fibula
Péroné *m*

Leg
Jambe *f*

Tarsus
Tarse *m*

Metatarsus
Métatarse *m*

Foot
Pied *m*

Toe
Orteil *m*

HADLEY PAGER INFO PUBLICATIONS
French-English, English-French

GLOSSARY OF HOUSE PURCHASE AND RENOVATION TERMS

Paperback, 2000, Fourth Edition, 56 pages, 210 x 148 mm
ISBN 1-872739-08-3   Price: £7.50
- Provides over 2000 French words and phrases used by estate agents, notaires, mortgage lenders, builders, decorators, etc.

GLOSSARY OF FRENCH LEGAL TERMS

Paperback, 1999, 114 pages, 210 x 148 mm
ISBN 1-872739-07-5   Price: £12.00
- Provides over 4000 French legal words and phrases associated with legislation falling within the Civil Code and the Penal Code, (eg house purchase and wills), but company and commercial legislation is not covered.

HADLEY'S CONVERSATIONAL FRENCH PHRASE BOOK

Paperback, 1997, 256 pages, 148 x 105 mm
ISBN 1-872739-05-9   Price: £6.00
- Over 2000 French/English phrases and 2000 English/French phrases
- Eleven conversational topic vocabularies
- Aide-memoire key word dictionary

GLOSSARY OF GARDENING AND HORTICULTURAL TERMS

Paperback, 2001, Second Edition, 68 pages, 210 x 148 mm
ISBN 1-872739-10-5   Price: £8.50
- The glossary includes around 1800 gardening and horticultural terms
- The glossary matches up the familiar French and English names of pot and garden flowering plants and shrubs which are not readily available elsewhere

HADLEY'S FRENCH MOTORING PHRASE BOOK & DICTIONARY

Paperback, 2001, 176 pages, 148 x 105 mm
ISBN 1-872739-09-1   Price: £6.00
- Asking the Way, Road Signs, Car Hire, Parking, Breakdowns, Accidents, Types of Vehicle, Cycling and Motor Sports. Extensive Dictionary
- Over 3000 words and phrases included

CONCISE DICTIONARY OF HOUSE BUILDING (Arranged by Trades)

Paperback, 2001, Second Edition, 256 pages, 210 x 144 mm
ISBN 1-872739-11-3   Price £27.00
- Dictionary is divided into 14 Sections covering various stages and trades employed in house building
- Over 10,000 terms in each language

The above publications are available through good booksellers or can be obtained directly from Hadley Pager Info by sending a cheque to cover the price (postage is free within the UK, add 10% if outside the UK) to **Hadley Pager Info, PO Box 249, Leatherhead, KT23 3WX, England**. Latest Publication List available on request.
Email: hpinfo@aol.com